THE NITRIC OXIDE (NO) SOLUTION

How to Boost the Body's Miracle Molecule to Prevent and Reverse Chronic Disease

by Nathan S. Bryan, PhD and Janet Zand, OMD
with Bill Gottlieb, CHC

Neogenis
248 Addie Roy Rd. Ste. B-201
Austin, Texas 78746
www.neogenis.com

© 2010 Neogenis

Recipes © 2010 Jennifer Adler, CN

Recipes, Raw Beet Salad and Fresh Green Cashew-Walnut Pate
© 2010 Janet Zand, OMD

ISBN: 978-0-615-41713-4

Cover design by Neogenis. Interior design by Sterling Hill Productions.
Packaged by Good For You Books

The information in this book is for educational purposes only. It is not intended to replace the
advice of a physician or medical practitioner. Please see your health care provider before beginning
any new health program.

CONTENTS

• PART ONE •

NO: The Body's Miracle Molecule

ONE

What Is NO?

*The Little-Known Key to Preventing
and Reversing Heart Disease*

Imagine for a moment a "miracle molecule" that could dramatically improve your health—*if* you could increase the amount of the molecule in your body.

Now, this molecule won't turn water into wine or raise anyone from the dead. It's not *that* kind of miraculous. But biologically speaking, it's definitely a miracle-maker. Because it can:

- prevent high blood pressure (hypertension), a disease that damages your heart, brain, and kidneys.
- keep your arteries young and flexible.
- prevent, slow, or reverse the buildup of artery-clogging arterial plaques.
- help stop the formation of artery-clogging blood clots—the result of plaques bursting and spilling their contents into the blood stream.
- lower cholesterol.
- by doing all of the above, reduce your risk of heart attack and stroke, the #1 and #3 killers of Americans.

But this molecule has more miracles to perform. It can also:

- reduce the risk of diabetes and disastrous diabetic complications, such as chronic kidney disease, blindness, hard-to-heal foot and leg ulcers, and amputations.
- limit the swelling and pain of arthritis, and boost the power of pain-relieving drugs.

- reverse erectile dysfunction (ED).
- calm the choking inflammation of asthma.
- protect your bones from osteoporosis.
- help provide the mood-lifting power behind antidepressant medications.
- assist the immune system in killing bacteria.
- limit skin damage from the sun.

"There may be no disease process where this miracle molecule does *not* have a protective role," we were told by Louis J. Ignarro, PhD, a 1998 Nobel Laureate. What is this miracle molecule?

Nitric oxide—otherwise known (by its chemical formula) as NO.

What Is Nitric Oxide?

What you're reading—right now—is a *signal*, a message, a communication that is moving from the page to your eyes and deep into your brain, where an energized collection of brain cells (neurons) makes sense out of it all. And that process happens *fast*—in nanoseconds, in less than the blink of an eye.

Nitric oxide (NO) works just like that.

Nitric oxide is a *signaling molecule*. A molecule, of course, is a combination of atoms, held together by electrical charges. Water is H_2O—two hydrogen atoms and one oxygen atom. Nitric oxide is NO—one atom of nitrogen and one atom of oxygen, as simple as can be. So simple, in fact, that it's a *gas*, not a liquid or solid.

When it's created and released, this gas easily and quickly penetrates nearby membranes and cells, sending its signals. In less than a second, NO signals:

- arteries to relax and expand.
- immune cells to kill bacteria and cancer cells.
- brain cells to communicate with each other.

Will the Real NO Please Stand Up?

It's easy to confuse NO (nitric oxide) with other, similarly named molecules.

It's not *nitrous oxide* (N_2O), the general anesthetic humorously known as laughing gas.

And it's not *nitrogen dioxide* (NO_2), an air pollutant formed from oxygen and NO.

It's just plain old NO—and it spells YES for health.

In fact, NO sends crucial signals within *every* cell, tissue, organ, and system of the body.

But perhaps its most important signaling function is within the circulatory system—the system that, in 21st-century America, so often goes wrong, triggering heart attacks and strokes.

Our Hurting Hearts

The stark statistics tell the story.

Eighty-one million American adults have cardiovascular disease (CVD)—one in three.

Every year, nearly one million people with CVD have their first heart attack. Of those, 141 thousand die.

In fact, CVD is the *leading* cause of death in the US, accounting for 36 percent of all deaths. If all forms of CVD were prevented, Americans would live an average of seven more years.

Another way to think of the nonstop tragedy of CVD: every 37 seconds (about the time it took you to read from the start of this section to the end of this sentence) another American dies of CVD.

It's time to say NO to CVD.

And to understand *how* NO works to protect you from CVD—the hardened, plaque-clogged arteries that lead to heart attacks and strokes—you have to understand how the *endothelium* works.

The biggest organ in your body—the endothelium

The endothelium is the *lining* of your blood vessels—*every* blood vessel, from the large coronary arteries of your heart to the tiny capillaries that transfer oxygen and nutrients from your bloodstream to your tissues. The endothelial lining is only one cell thick, but that's still a lot of cells: if you took all the endothelial cells in your body and laid them out on a flat surface, they'd cover a soccer field.

To get a better view of the endothelium, let's zoom in on a coronary artery. In a healthy artery, the endothelium is smooth and blood flows freely. The artery is also flexible (as compared to a "hardened" artery affected by heart disease): it easily widens, or dilates, a function medical experts call *vasodilation*.

Zoom in even closer, and we find out that NO is manufactured *in* the endothelium, via several different biochemical pathways. (You'll read more about them in Chapter 3.)

In one pathway, the amino acid *L-arginine* (a component of protein foods such as meat, fish, dairy, beans, and nuts) combines with oxygen to produce NO. This process is sparked by three enzymes collectively called *nitric oxide synthase* (NOS). One of those enzymes—endothelial nitric oxide synthase, or eNOS—starts the activation of NO in the endothelium. NO is also produced directly from the chemical compounds nitrate and nitrite.

But no matter the pathway, the end result is the creation of the molecule that has been dubbed the "endothelium-derived relaxing factor."

Why that name?

Because NO diffuses out of the endothelium into a layer beneath it, the *smooth muscle* of the artery. There, it signals the muscles to *relax*—to widen, to expand, to undergo *vasodilation*.

Needless to say, vasodilation increases blood flow—instead of a measly trickle, there's a steady and health-giving current of nutrient- and oxygen-rich blood circulating throughout your body.

What if you don't have enough NO?

Well, the opposite of a relaxed, widened artery is a tense, tightened artery—and when blood flows through that smaller space, blood pressure rises. Without enough NO, in other words, you develop high blood pressure, or hypertension—a major risk factor for heart disease and stroke, as the increased pressure damages artery walls, setting the stage for artery-clogging plaques to grow. (For more about the progression of heart disease, see the box "The Many Steps of Cardiovascular Disease" on pages 6–7.)

But NO does much more to protect the heart than regulate blood pressure.

If there's too little NO:

- Two of the building blocks of plaque (the white blood cells of the immune system and the tiny, plate-shaped blood factors called platelets) become glue-like, stick to the endothelium, and start the buildup of plaque.
- The smooth muscle cells of the artery wall start multiplying, growing into plaque.
- There's more chronic inflammation and oxidation in the arteries—the two driving forces of CVD.

Chronic inflammation is a low-grade version of the same redness, heat, and swelling that occur when the immune system rushes to a cut to stop infection.

Oxidation is what happens when a sliced apple turns brown or a chunk of iron rusts—only now it's happening to your cells.

- Inflammation and oxidation (also called *oxidative stress*) damage arterial cells, promoting plaque. Once plaque is formed, inflammation and oxidation destabilize plaque: it can burst open, spilling out the toxic contents that trigger artery-plugging blood clots.
- There's also more risk of the condition called *sudden cardiac death* (SCD). In more than 50 percent of people with heart disease, a sudden, unpredicted, deadly heart attack is the *first sign* of heart disease—and endothelial dysfunction (and low NO) plays a key role.

As you can see, the low-NO process *is* the process of CVD. And it's also a vicious cycle: the high blood pressure, chronic inflammation, and

The Many Steps of Cardiovascular Disease

Cardiovascular disease—the arterial damage that leads to a heart attack or stroke—is a step-by-step process that starts with damage to the endothelium. Here are the steps:

1. The endothelial lining of the artery is damaged—by high blood pressure, cigarette smoke, saturated fat, or other factors.
2. "Bad" LDL cholesterol becomes wedged in the damaged lining.
3. The LDL cholesterol starts to oxidize, the same way fat becomes rancid.
4. The endothelial cells release chemicals that tell the immune system that damage has occurred.
5. The immune system sends white blood cells called monocytes to the area of the injury—an inflammatory process (like immune cells rushing to the site of a cut to prevent infection, causing heat and redness).
6. The monocytes stick to the endothelium.
7. The endothelial cells release *more* distress signals, turning the monocytes into macrophages, cells that can engulf and dissolve foreign invaders such as viruses and bacteria.
8. But the macrophages *don't* dissolve the LDL—instead, they get stuck in it.
9. The macrophages then send out their distress signals, like a sergeant calling for more troops; new white blood cells arrive—but they also get stuck.

oxidation of the plaque-making process *further* decrease your ability to make NO, leading to more CVD, leading to less NO, leading to more CVD, and so on, and on.

The discovery of NO

A series of scientific discoveries in the 1970s and 1980s led to the discovery that won three scientists the Nobel Prize in 1998: NO is *the* compound manufactured by the endothelium to relax and dilate arteries.

Since that time, there has been an explosion of research about NO and

10. This is the beginning of *arterial plaque*—a fatty steak of oxidized LDL and dead macrophages.
11. As the plaque continues to accumulate, inflammation-making immune factors called cytokines send out signals that attract more immune cells, increasing the buildup.
12. The plaque also attracts other substances that the body typically sends to the site of an infection, such as fibrinogen (a protein that helps clot blood) and C-reactive protein (a biomarker of inflammation that is now acknowledged as a risk factor for heart disease).
13. Plaque breeds plaque: the inflamed area also inflames nearby cells, starting the plaque-producing process in those spots.
14. To protect itself, the body seals off a lump of plaque with a hard "cap" composed of the proteins collagen and elastin.
15. Beneath the cap, dead cells decay and pus builds up.
16. The fibrous cap can stay in place. But it can also thin and rupture, spilling pus and other toxins into the artery—triggering the artery-plugging blood clots that cause most heart attacks and strokes.

Having plenty of NO on hand can *prevent* this step-by-step process from starting ... *slow* the process if it starts ... or *reverse* the process if low levels of NO are restored to normal.

its many functions—more than 100 thousand scientific studies. Some key and interesting findings about NO:

The three little enzymes. NO production is triggered by three *enzymes*, proteins that spark chemical reactions. In the brain, it's neuronal nitric oxide synthase—nNOS, or NOSI. In the immune system, it's inducible nitric oxide synthase—iNOS, or NOSII. In the endothelium, it's endothelial nitric oxide synthase—eNOS, or NOSIII.

Nitroglycerin works via NO. We now understand that this old and effective treatment for angina (chest pain from narrowed arteries) works because it is transformed into nitrite, which is converted to artery-relaxing NO in the body.

Viagra depends on NO. Viagra and other medicines for erectile dysfunction (ED) work because they improve NO signaling in the penis.

Tibetans have 100 times more NO-forming nitrate and nitrite in their blood than people living at sea level. It dilates their arteries, helping them cope with the low levels of oxygen at high altitudes.

Plants produce NO, too. The molecule protects plant cells from cellular oxidation and disease.

But the most important discovery about NO has been its role in protecting you against CVD.

The Scientific Proof for the Artery-Protecting Power of NO

Hundreds of studies have been conducted demonstrating the artery-protecting power of NO. We report a few of them here to help convince you of the utter importance of maintaining or boosting levels of this molecule in your body.

(In Chapter 2, we discuss other diseases that can be prevented or treated by NO. And in Chapters 3, 4, and 5 we discuss the how-to of boosting blood and tissue levels of NO.)

Remember as you read these studies: where there's smoke, there's fire— and where there is what doctors call *endothelial dysfunction*, there is a deficiency of NO.

Endothelial dysfunction predicts heart disease. Researchers at the National Institutes of Health (NIH) conducted a type of study you'll read a lot about in this book: they injected the artery-dilating compound *acetylcholine* into an artery of study participants and measured how much the brachial artery of the forearm widened (dilated). This is a standard method for testing endothelial health (or the lack of it).

In a study of 308 people—176 with coronary artery disease (CAD) and 132 without it—the researchers measured endothelial function and then followed the study participants for the next four years, tracking "acute unpredictable cardiovascular events"—hard-to-control (unstable) angina, heart attacks, strokes, and deaths from cardiovascular disease.

Among those with *and* without heart disease, endothelial function was an accurate predictor of who did and didn't have a cardiovascular event. Those with a well-functioning endothelium (a sign of normal levels of NO) were unlikely to have a cardiovascular event; those with a weak endothelium (a sign of low levels of NO) were likely to have them. The findings were in the medical journal *Circulation*.

In a similar study in *Circulation*, Italian researchers tested the endothelial function of 42 women with chest pain but arteries that appeared normal when they were injected with dye and x-rayed (angiography).

Over 10 years, those who had vasodilation in response to an acetylcholine injection (a sign of a healthy endothelium and normal levels of NO) had "complete resolution" of their chest pain.

In contrast, of those who had *vasoconstriction* in response to the injection, one died and 13 continued to complain of chest pain—and a second angiography showed the development of CAD.

"Endothelial dysfunction in a setting of normal coronary arteries is a sign of future development of atherosclerosis," concluded the researchers.

And a review of studies on endothelial function and heart disease by a team of researchers from the Mayo Clinic College of Medicine showed that people with endothelial dysfunction had:

- more heart attacks.
- more need for surgery to open clogged arteries.
- more deaths from heart disease.

These studies, they concluded, "underscore the systemic nature of endothelial dysfunction and its pivotal role in prediction of cardiovascular events."

Less NO, less endothelial repair. In an animal study, researchers found that low levels of NO impaired the number and function of *endothelial progenitor cells*—cells that are responsible for maintaining and repairing the endothelium.

High fat, low NO. How many times have you heard—from the press, from your doctor, from your spouse—that eating less saturated fat can help you avoid heart disease? We'd guess a lot of times. But those folks probably didn't tell that you one of the main reasons *why* a high-fat meal hurts your heart is because it decreases your NO. Case in point:

Researchers in the Department of Cardiology at the University of Maryland School of Medicine studied two groups of students. One group ate a fast-food breakfast containing 900 calories and 50 grams of fat; the other group ate the same amount of calories for breakfast, but no fat. After the meals, the researchers measured vasodilation—and found that vasodilation in those who ate the high-fat meal was dramatically decreased for the next four hours!

(In a similar study, the same researchers found that giving people two antioxidant vitamins before the fatty meal—1,000 mg of vitamin C and 800 IU of vitamin E—prevented the decrease in vasodilation. Those results were in the *Journal of the American Medical Association*.)

More risk factors for heart disease, less NO. Nearly every risk factor for heart disease—high blood pressure, high "bad" LDL cholesterol, high total cholesterol, low "good" HDL cholesterol, high triglycerides (a blood fat that can hurt the heart), diabetes (which dramatically increases the risk of heart attack and stroke), cigarette smoking, physical inactivity, high levels of the amino acid homocysteine, and aging (discussed later in this chapter)—*also* causes endothelial dysfunction and low levels of NO.

Why?

One probable reason: all those factors *increase* the compound *asymmetric dimethylarginine* (ADMA). This chemical shoves aside L-arginine—blocking the production of the NO-generating enzyme NOS, and therefore blocking the production of NO.

Another reason: those factors also increase oxidative stress, which quickly inactivates NO after it's produced.

Over-40 Arteries Need More NO

There are many risk factors for heart disease. High blood pressure. High cholesterol. A mom or a dad (or both) who died of heart disease.

African-Americans and NO

Compared to whites, African-Americans have more high blood pressure, heart disease, and heart failure (a weakened heart muscle that doesn't pump as much blood); develop those problems earlier in life; and die more often from heart disease. One statistic makes the point: a black man who is 45 to 65 years old is *four times* more likely to have a stroke than a white man of the same age.

Obviously, there are many reasons for differences in CVD between blacks and whites, including socioeconomic and other factors. But one important reason may be that African-Americans tend to produce less NO.

Healthy and hypertensive blacks have more endothelial dysfunction than healthy and hypertensive whites—a sure sign of a deficiency of NO.

A genetic variation (polymorphism) in eNOS that may block the production of NO is more common in African-Americans.

A deficiency of another enzyme that plays a role in the creation of NO (glucose-6-phosphate dehydrogenase, or G6PD) is very common among African-Americans—and studies show that this deficiency impairs endothelial function and vasodilation.

And in a study called the "African-American Heart Failure Trial," those who used a drug that may improve nitric oxide production —isosorbide dinitrate combined with hydralazine (BiDil)—had a 39 percent lower rate of hospitalization and a 43 percent lower death rate than those taking a placebo.

Our conclusion: if you're African-American, think very seriously about natural ways to boost NO, such as those discussed in this book.

But one risk factor that is common to *everybody* who reaches age 40 is . . . reaching age 40. Yes, aging—all by itself—is a risk factor for a heart attack or stroke. Why?

Aging leads to an accumulation of protein in artery walls, making them stiffer. With aging, you have fewer capillaries, the tiniest, cell-wide blood vessels. But perhaps most importantly, as you age, so does your endothelium: you don't generate as much NO, and your arteries don't dilate as easily and as widely. They're narrow. They're stiff. They're a setup for a heart attack or stroke.

A couple of studies graphically demonstrate the effect of aging on your endothelium.

The older you are, the weaker your endothelium—because of less NO

In one study, Italian researchers evaluated forearm blood flow—the standard measurement of endothelial health—in 47 people with normal blood pressure and 49 people with high blood pressure. They found that in *both* groups, those who were older had poorer endothelial-dependent vasodilation: the NO-sparked ability of arteries to widen and permit health-giving blood flow. And that weakening of the endothelium was in perfect parallel to aging—decade by decade, NO-powered, endothelial-dependent vasodilation decreased. Specifically:

30 years old and younger. Endothelial-dependent vasodilation was strongest.

31 to 45 years old. Vasodilation was 11 percent weaker than in the 30-and-younger set.

46 to 60 years old. Vasodilation was 13 percent weaker than in the 31- to 45-year-olds.

60 and older. Vasodilation was 28 percent weaker than in the 46- to 60-year-olds.

All in all, those 60 and older had vasodilation that was 52 percent weaker—less than *half* as strong—as those 30 and younger. And these were older people who did *not* have high blood pressure!

"Advancing age is an independent factor leading to the progressive impairment of endothelium-dependent vasodilation in humans," concluded the researchers in the journal *Circulation*.

Why does the endothelium weaken with age?

"A progressive reduction of NO availability," wrote the researchers. In fact, they wrote, their findings suggest that "in aged individuals NO availability is *almost totally compromised.*" (Emphasis ours.)

In a similar study, Japanese researchers tested vasodilation in 18 healthy people, aged 23 to 70. A list of the patients and their response to the vasodilator is striking, showing a near-perfect correlation between age and endothelial health.

The 23-year-old in the study had an artery that expanded more than *five times* its width when the individual was given a vasodilator; the artery of the 70-year-old expanded a little more than *two times*.

"Coronary blood flow response to acetylcholine (an endothelium-dependent vasodilator) decreased significantly with aging," concluded the researchers in the journal *Circulation*.

Why?

Probably because of the age-related decrease in the release of "endothelium-derived relaxing factor"—a scientific name for NO.

Another study by the same team of Japanese researchers found a loss of 75 percent of endothelium-produced NO in people 70 to 80 years old as compared to 20-year-olds.

It's important to emphasize that this decline happens not only to people with CVD but to *healthy* older adults: people who *don't* have high blood pressure . . . people who *don't* have high cholesterol . . . people who *don't* have circulation-damaging diabetes.

In other words, it happens to everybody who gets older!

But don't despair.

All of these studies also show that the ability of arteries to *widen* didn't change—just the ability of the endothelium to generate artery-widening NO.

And there are plenty of ways to generate more NO, as you'll read about in Chapters 3, 4, and 5: a diet rich in NO-producing nitrate and nitrite (mainly from leafy greens); an NO-boosting supplement; NO-restoring regular exercise; and lifestyle factors that preserve and increase NO, such as sufficient sleep and stress control.

The age-related decrease of NO is *not* inevitable.

You can slow down the loss of NO.

You can stop the loss of NO.

You can reverse the loss of NO.

That's what the rest of this book shows you how to do.

TWO

NO vs. Disease

NO Contest!

Cardiovascular disease (CVD)—the heart attacks, strokes, and heart failure that kill most Americans—isn't the only health problem that NO can help prevent, slow, or reverse.

"NO, generated by eNOS and nNOS [two enzymes that spark the production of NO], plays a ubiquitous role in the body in controlling the function of almost every, if not every, organ system," is the way a team of scientists at Pennington Biomedical Research Center in Louisiana summed up the situation, in the medical journal *Experimental Gerontology*.

In other words, in your immune system . . . in the hormone-generating glands of your endocrine system . . . in your digestive system . . . in your respiratory system . . . in the brain and spinal cord of your central nervous system—in "almost every, if not every, organ system," as those researchers put it—NO is hard at work, protecting and restoring your health.

So it's no surprise that a huge (and growing) body of scientific literature (more than 100 thousand studies, some of them in a medical journal called *Nitric Oxide* that is devoted solely to the molecule) describes the many roles that NO plays and also *might* play in health and healing.

We say "might" because the fact that NO is a crucial signaling molecule in every organ is a relatively recent discovery, and scientists are still working out *exactly* how NO works to maintain health and heal the body. (And the role of NO in healing depends on "just right" amounts: as we describe in Chapter 6, too *much* NO can harm the body, like any other compound.)

In this chapter, we're taking you on a guided tour through the highlights of the scientific literature on the role of NO in disease prevention and cure. The reason we're presenting so much scientific evidence about NO and disease: we want to make the very important point—again and again—that this miracle molecule really *is* miraculous, with the power to positively affect "almost every, if not every, organ system."

Let's start with your bones . . .

Arthritis: Do Painkillers Work Better with NO?

In osteoarthritis, the cartilage that cushions bones wears away, the bones painfully rub together, and the structures around the joint—the tendons, ligaments, and muscles—become strained, inflamed, and painful. Osteoarthritis affects 27 million Americans, and is the #1 cause of disability in the US. (Rheumatoid arthritis is an autoimmune disease, in which the immune system mistakenly attacks the joints; it affects 2.5 million Americans. This section will focus on osteoarthritis, calling it just "arthritis.")

The type of drug most people take to deal with the chronic pain of arthritis are the nonsteroidal anti-inflammatory drugs, or NSAIDs. There are dozens of such drugs, but some of the more common ones include ibuprofen (Advil, Motrin), naproxen (Aleve, Naprosyn), and diclofenac (Voltaren, Cataflam).

But like any drug, NSAIDs have several downsides—including the fact that they can kill you. This was revealed when it was discovered that the new generation of NSAIDs—the so-called COX-2 inhibitors, such as celecoxib (Celebrex), and the now-banned valdecoxib (Bextra) and rofecoxib (Vioxx)—raised blood pressure and the risk of heart attack and stroke. (Some experts estimate the drugs killed at least 150 thousand people before they were pulled from the market.) In the wake of that pharmaceutical massacre, researchers turned their attention to the entire class of NSAIDs—and found that ibuprofen, naproxen, and diclofenac also increase your risk of heart attack and stroke.

That's the bad news. The good news: taking an NO-increasing supplement *with* those drugs may help prevent the problem.

The French NO-connection
In fact, a French pharmaceutical company created a NSAID that also boosted levels of NO: naproxcinod, intended to prevent the rise of blood pressure and the risk of CVD with NSAIDs. To test the drug, doctors from

the Northwestern University Feinberg School of Medicine conducted a 13-week study, giving nearly one thousand people with arthritis either naproxcinod, Aleve, or a placebo. Naproxcinod relieved the pain and symptoms of arthritis as well as Aleve and better than the placebo. But, unlike Aleve, naproxcinod *didn't* increase blood pressure.

"These results demonstrated the clinical efficacy and safety of naproxcinod in the management of the signs and symptoms of osteoarthritis," concluded the researchers in the May 2010 issue of the medical journal *Osteoarthritis and Cartilage*. "Naproxcinod was well-tolerated, with blood pressure effects similar to placebo and different from naproxen."

But in May 2010, the FDA declined to approve the drug, asking the company for more safety data.

Our perspective: if you're taking a NSAID for arthritis, you should talk to your doctor about also taking an NO-boosting supplement, which we discuss in Chapter 3. (An additional bonus: that NO-boosting supplement may also help protect you from stomach ulcers, which yearly kill 16,500 NSAID-takers, and hospitalize another 200 thousand. You'll read more about the ulcer-stopping powers of NO later in this chapter.)

And that supplement might not only prevent side effects—it also might help some NSAIDs work better to relieve pain.

Ibuprofen works better with NO

In an animal study, combining ibuprofen with NO-boosting L-arginine increased the anti-inflammatory power of the drug, reported Italian researchers from the University of Milano.

"NO may limit inflammation . . . and anti-inflammatory compounds able to release NO display higher efficacy," they concluded in the journal *Pharmacological Research*.

Their suggestion: if you have arthritis, take an anti-inflammatory drug *and* take an NO-boosting supplement to "exploit the beneficial effects of NO."

More NO, less arthritis pain

Other researchers have found NO reduces arthritis pain on its own.

In a study in the *Clinical Journal of Pain*, researchers from the Physical

Therapy Program at the University of Colorado–Denver theorized that NO is a key factor in the reduction of arthritis pain.

They hypothesized that NO is decreased in joints stressed by "chronic load-induced stress" (such as knee arthritis in people who are overweight) and "biochemical change-induced stresses" (such as the oxidative damage in bones caused by diets high in saturated fat and low in antioxidant-rich vegetables and fruits).

Based on the fact that NO is decreased in arthritis, the researchers speculated that "NO-based intervention may produce substantial pain relief without undesirable side effects, by increasing circulation, decreasing nerve irritation, and decreasing inflammation in joints."

Their conclusion: NO "can bring dramatic relief to people with painful osteoarthritis."

Aging: If You're Over 40, You Probably Need More NO

It's a frustrating fact of life: as you age, your endothelium ages with you, and your production of NO drops year by year by year. That's the reason cardiovascular disease is far more common among senior citizens than seniors in college.

The aging circulatory system, wrote a team of Spanish researchers in the journal *Ageing Research Reviews*, has a deteriorating balance between artery-expanding and artery-tightening compounds, and this is "mainly characterized by a progressive reduction of the bioavailability of NO."

Why does NO decline?

Endothelial cells age, wrote the researchers. Damage from oxidative stress builds up. The aging immune system can't keep cell-damaging compounds (cytokines) under control. The genes of aging kick in. And because of these changes, boosting your NO through diet and exercise may become less effective.

That's one of the reasons why, if you're 40 years old or older, we strongly recommend you consider a NO-boosting supplement to make up the shortfall in your body's ability to generate artery-saving NO. This is particularly important if your blood pressure is higher than 130/80 mm Hg—the incontestable sign of a damaged endothelium and NO deficiency.

Altitude Sickness: Preventing Disease at 7,000 Feet

Altitude sickness—formally called *acute mountain sickness* (AMS)—affects about 50 percent of people who travel from their homes at or near sea level to a destination at 7,000 feet or higher, such as Mexico City or Aspen, Colorado.

Its cause: the body doesn't have enough time to adapt to the lower levels of oxygen in the atmosphere at that altitude. Typical symptoms include headaches and nausea for a day or two. But a very small percentage of people with AMS go on to develop a life-threatening respiratory problem called high altitude pulmonary edema (HAPE), in which the alveoli—the tiny structures that pass oxygen from the lungs into the bloodstream—fill up with fluid.

Writing in the journal *Progress in Cardiovascular Diseases*, a team of Swiss doctors from the Botnar Center for Extreme Medicine theorized that "impaired . . . epithelial NO synthesis and/or bioavailability" is the "central underlying defect" that predisposes some people to develop HAPE.

Our advice: if you're planning to travel to an altitude higher than 7,000 feet, talk to your doctor about taking an NO-boosting supplement to help prevent AMS and HAPE.

(You can read more about NO and high-altitude living—showing that Tibetans living at high altitudes have more than *ten* times the level of NO as Americans living at sea level—on page 91 of Chapter 4.)

Asthma: Opening Closed Airways with NO

Twenty-seven million American children and adults have asthma: inflamed, constricted, mucous-clogged airways (bronchi), with symptoms such as wheezing, shortness of breath, coughing, phlegm, and chest tightness. The number of people with asthma has quadrupled in the last three decades—and the number of deaths from asthma (caused by a bronchi-shutting severe asthma attack) has doubled.

Experts speculate the causes of that increase include: more allergens (many people with asthma also have allergies, which trigger asthma attacks); higher levels of air pollution, outdoors and in; an inflammation-causing diet high in saturated fat and refined carbohydrates and low in vegetables, fruits, fish, whole grains, and beans; and higher levels of stress (which causes the chronic release of cortisol, an inflammation-increasing hormone).

How can NO help?

As you've learned, NO sends a signal for blood vessels to *dilate*—to widen. Well, it can also help widen so-called "hyperresponsive" airways that react to an allergen, pollutant, or other trigger by tightening and turning breathing into a wheeze.

Boosting NO, relieving asthma

In a study of animals with experimentally induced asthma, researchers found a "deficiency of bronchodilating nitric oxide (NO)" and increased "airway hyperresponsiveness."

They also found that giving animals NO-boosting L-arginine "reverses allergen-induced hyperresponsiveness." The findings were in the *American Journal of Respiratory and Critical Care Medicine*.

Treating asthma with NO

Writing in the *European Journal of Pharmacology*, researchers from the Department of Respiratory Medicine at Hammersmith Hospital in London observed that NO plays a "homeostatic bronchoprotective role [maintains biochemical balance in the airways]" and might be used to treat inflammatory airway diseases such as asthma.

And in a paper titled "Nitric Oxide in asthma therapy," a team of Dutch researchers list the "potential protective effects of nitric oxide" in asthma, including:

- calming nerves that tighten airways.
- relaxing muscles.

- making airways less hyperresponsive to bronchi-tightening triggers.
- calming the immune system so it doesn't overreact to asthma triggers.

"It is likely that new developments in this area [using NO to treat asthma] will drastically change respiratory medicine during the coming 5 to 10 years," the researchers concluded in the journal *Current Pharmaceutical Design*.

Bladder Problems

Urinary incontinence, bladder infections, and other bladder problems affect millions of people (most of them women). NO may help.

Researchers from the Wake Forest Institute for Regenerative Medicine observed that NO relaxes the muscles of the urethra (the tube that empties the bladder), and might also play a role in the ability to control the detrusor muscle (which contracts while urinating).

In an animal study, the researchers found that mice bred to have bladder dysfunction also had "low bioavailable NO." The findings were in the *Journal of Urology*.

Cancer: Improving Treatment with NO

Cancer is notoriously difficult to treat because of two main factors, observed a team of Belgian researchers in a review paper on cancer and nitric oxide in the *European Journal of Cancer*: (1) hypoxia, the lack of oxygen in and around the tumor; (2) the variable levels of blood flow to the tumor.

But NO can help "circumvent these sources of resistance" to cancer therapy, they wrote. NO can also "sensitize" the tumor to treatment with chemotherapy and radiation. Specifically, NO can:

- alter blood flow to improve the effectiveness of drug therapy (so-called *provascular* treatment).

- sensitize cancer cells to radiation.
- limit DNA damage from radiation.
- boost the cancer-killing ability of macrophages (immune cells).

"Exploitation of the biology of NO offers the opportunity to improve the efficacy of conventional anticancer treatments such as chemo- and radiotherapy," concluded the researchers.

Chronic Obstructive Pulmonary Disease (COPD): Treating Breathlessness with NO

Everybody knows that smoking causes lung cancer. It also causes chronic obstructive pulmonary disease, or COPD (either emphysema, chronic bronchitis, or both), the fourth leading cause of death in the US, killing more people than diabetes, Alzheimer's, the flu, or accidents.

The main treatment for COPD: drugs that improve lung function and ease breathlessness. And they may work by boosting NO.

Finnish researchers studied 40 people with COPD before and after treating with COPD drugs—and those who had the biggest improvement in lung function and the biggest decrease in breathlessness also had "high levels of bronchial NO flux," reported the researchers in the *European Respiratory Journal*.

Dementia: Normal NO, Normal Brain

The brain depends on NO. The enzyme nNOS—neuronal nitric oxide synthase—makes sure the brain is well-supplied with this signaling molecule, which helps brain cells communicate with each other, and keeps them in a balanced state (rather than the "excitotoxicity" caused by overactive neurons).

But with aging, a lot of brains stop working.

Nearly five million Americans suffer from dementia, in most cases either

Alzheimer's disease (caused by a buildup of toxic proteins in the brain) or vascular dementia (caused by a stroke or other circulatory problems). Problems with NO may play a role.

"Abnormal NO signaling could . . . contribute to a variety of neurodegenerative pathologies, such as . . . Alzheimer's disease," concluded a team of UK researchers in a scientific paper on NO and the brain in the journal *The Neuroscientist*. Other research supports their statement.

Animals with dementia have low NO

In a study of experimental animals bred to have dementia-like brain changes early in life, Chinese researchers found that "downregulation [poor production] of NO" might cause the learning and memory problems in the animals. The findings were in the *International Journal of Neuroscience*.

Ditto for people with dementia

Spanish researchers tested the blood levels of NO in 99 people with dementia and 55 people of a similar age without the disease—and found "a significant decrease of . . . NO levels in dementia, especially in . . . Alzheimer's disease and vascular dementia patients, as compared" with the non-dementia group. They also found a link between lower NO levels and a greater degree of "cognitive deterioration" in those with dementia.

"Our data suggest that low NO may contribute to the pathogenesis [development] of dementia," concluded the researchers in the journal *Neuroscience Letters*.

Diabetes: Sugar-Regulating Insulin Needs NO

Type 2 diabetes—fasting blood sugar (glucose) levels above 125 mg/dL—is an epidemic in America, affecting 24 million Americans, more than half of them over 60. Another 57 million Americans have prediabetes: fasting blood sugar levels 100 to 125 mg/dL.

High blood sugar slowly but surely destroys the circulatory system—every inch of it. High blood sugar:

- quadruples the risk of heart disease and stroke.
- is one of the leading causes of kidney disease, an organ rich in blood vessels (diabetic nephropathy).
- destroys blood vessels in the eye, and is the leading cause of blindness (diabetic retinopathy).
- cuts off circulation to the nerves, causing burning pain and numbness (diabetic neuropathy).
- creates skin ulcers that won't heal (diabetic ulcers), leading to amputations of toes, feet, and legs. (Diabetes is the #1 cause of nontraumatic amputation of lower limbs.)
- more than doubles the risk of Alzheimer's disease.
- Needless to say, it also shortens life: a diagnosis of diabetes in a 40-year-old man shortens his life expectancy by 10 years; in a 40-year-old woman, by 12 years. (And in today's diabetes epidemic, it's not unusual for *children* to be diagnosed with type 2 diabetes.)

Low NO may play a key role in the development of type 2 diabetes.

Insulin needs NO

Your body regulates blood sugar levels with the hormone insulin, which ushers glucose out of the bloodstream and into cells. In fact, prediabetes is also called *insulin resistance*: the insulin receptors on cells no longer respond to the hormone, like locks that can't use a key.

"NO regulates insulin signaling and secretion," wrote a team of Irish researchers in a paper (in the journal *Clinical Science*) that explored why exercise can help prevent diabetes. (For much more information on exercise and NO, please see Chapter 4.)

"NO synthesis is essential for glucose uptake," they continued.

"If levels of NO are decreased, insulin resistance will result," they added.

Diabetes decreases NOS

Writing in the journal *Clinical Science*, doctors from the Cardiovascular Research Institute at Maastricht University Medical Center in the

Netherlands noted that there is a "diabetes-induced impairment of eNOS"—one of the enzymes that sparks the production of NO.

In an experiment to prove the point, researchers from the Division of Endocrinology, Diabetes, and Metabolism at the Cleveland Clinic found that insulin sparked a twofold increase in NOS activity in healthy people—but no increase in NOS in people with type 2 diabetes. The findings were in the journal *Metabolic Syndromes and Related Disorders*.

Less NO, less blood flow

Similarly, a team of Japanese researchers, writing in the journal *Pharmacology and Therapeutics*, noted that "reduced NOS expression and activity and/or NO availability" interferes with blood flow in diabetes—in "the brain, eye, heart, kidney, skeletal muscle, skin, and penile tissues."

AGEs reduce NO

AGEs is an acronym for *advanced glycation end products*—a warping of a protein (such as the collagen in skin) or a fat (such as the membranes of brain cells) when excess glucose binds to them.

The more AGEs, the more risk of chronic disease—and, needless to say, people with diabetes and chronically high blood sugar have more AGEs.

When Australian researchers injected experimental animals with AGEs, they found much lower levels of nitric oxide production. "We demonstrate that AGEs represent a potentially important cause of vascular dysfunction, linked to the induction of nitric oxide resistance," concluded the researchers in the *Journal of Hypertension*.

More NO, better healing for diabetic foot ulcers

"Nitric oxide deficiency has been established as an important mechanism responsible for poor wound healing in diabetic foot ulcer patients," observed researchers from the Wound Healing Center at Virginia Commonwealth University in Richmond, in the *Journal of Wound Ostomy and Continence Nursing*.

(In a study in the journal *Molecular Pharmacology*, researchers at the University of Toronto revealed that they had created a new "NO-delivery platform" for a bandage to be used in the healing of diabetic foot ulcers, and had tested it successfully in animal experiments.)

The bottom line seems obvious to us: if you want to prevent prediabetes or diabetes, or lessen the risk of its circulation-destroying complications— increase NO.

Erectile Dysfunction: When NO Means Yes

New research shows that erectile dysfunction (ED) is an early warning sign of cardiovascular disease (CVD): in a 10-year study, guys who had ED at the start of the study were 80 percent more likely to develop CVD by the study's end.

Yes, ED is usually a *circulatory* problem—lack of blood flow to the penis. And that's why NO helps.

Drugs such as sildenafil (Viagra), vardenafil (Levitra), and tadalafil (Cialis) all work with the same mechanism: they let NO go to work and stay at work. Here's the step-by-step process:

1. NO binds to the receptors of an enzyme called guanylyl cyclase.
2. This boosts levels of a compound called cGMP (cyclic guanosine monophosphate), which leads to widening of the arteries in the penis.
3. More blood flows into the penis, filling the corpus cavernosum, the spongy tissue that expands to form an erection.
4. Viagra and other ED drugs work by blocking the compound PDE5 (phosphodiesterase type 5), which dissolves cGMP.

We won't cite a bunch of scientific studies proving that Viagra, Levitra, and Cialis work. Watch just about any sporting event on TV and you'll hear a lot of middle-aged male actors attesting to the effectiveness of these drugs.

Eye Disease: Can You Read the N and the O?

The following scientific statement may not be an example of easy-to-read prose, but it makes one thing perfectly clear: your eyes need NO.

"NO is an important mediator of homeostatic [health-giving, disease-preventing] processes in the eye, such as regulation of aqueous humor dynamics [the amount of fluid inside the eyeball], retinal neurotransmission [the role of the retina in sending electrical signals to the brain] and phototransduction [the conversion of light into electrical signal]," noted a team of French researchers in the journal *Survey of Ophthalmology*.

That's why "underproduction of NO results in various eye diseases," wrote a team of eye doctors from the Institute of Ocular Pharmacology at the Texas A&M University System Health Science Center, in the *Journal of Ocular Pharmacology and Therapeutics*.

And those diseases "could be corrected by providing NOS substrates or NO donors to lower intraocular pressure [preventing and treating glaucoma], increase ocular blood flow [preventing and treating age-related macular degeneration], etc.," the researchers continued.

"Underexpression of NO could contribute to pathological conditions of the eye," agreed Italian researchers from the Medical School of the University of Catania, in the medical journal *Drug News and Perspectives*. "From a clinical perspective," they continued, "precise regulation of NO may lead to new therapeutic options likely safer and more efficacious than currently available treatments for various sight-threatening eye diseases."

NO for glaucoma

In a study in the journal *Oftalmologia*, a team of Hungarian researchers reported that they observed important, vision-regulating NO activity in the eyes of people with glaucoma (damage to the optic nerve and to vision caused by high levels of "intraocular" pressure within the eyeball)—a finding that "suggests an important role of NO in future therapies for glaucoma."

How might NO work to treat glaucoma?

The high level of pressure is caused by a clogged "trabecular meshwork"—an area that drains fluid from the eye. "The increase of NO increases vasodilation [widening of blood vessels] and improves contractility in the trabecular meshwork, the final effect being the decrease of intraocular pressure," wrote the researchers.

Infections: Bacteria Are No Match for NO

NO is generated by two immune cells as part of their bacteria- and virus-killing process: by macrophages, amoeba-like white blood cells that engulf and dissolve bacteria, viruses, and other invaders; and by neutrophils, white blood cells that race to the site of any invasion, injury, or other disturbance to begin the healing process.

The NO in these cells is generated by the enzyme iNOS—inducible nitric oxide synthase.

At the first biochemical sign of infection or injury—the production of immune compounds called cytokines—iNOS gets busy, generating germ-killing NO within two to four hours.

Bacteria-beating NO

In a study by researchers in the Department of Chemistry and Biochemistry at the University of California–Santa Cruz, published in the journal *ACS Medicinal Chemistry Letters*, an NO-boosting device killed several types of bacteria, including:

- *Pseudomonas aeruginosa* (a common bacteria that can cause many types of infections, including "hot tub rash")
- *Escherichia coli* (the bacteria that causes many cases of food poisoning)
- *Staphylococcus aureus* (the most common cause of staph infections, such as boils and rashes)
- methicillin-resistant *Staphylococcus aureus* (MRSA, the antibiotic-resistant bacteria running rampant in American hospitals)

Insomnia: Senior Sleepers Nod Off with NO

Fifty-eight percent of adults age 59 and over report having difficulty sleeping at least a few nights a week. The cause might be too little NO.

REM sleep needs NO

Rapid eye movement (REM) sleep occurs during dreaming—and REM sleep begins to decline during aging.

In animal experiments, a team of French researchers found that "NO derived from iNOS" triggers and maintains REM sleep during aging. The findings were in the journal *Neurobiology of Aging*.

Losing sleep? Find NO.

When you lose sleep—after staying up late studying or working, for example—your body tries to recover by sleeping more.

In an animal experiment, a team of Finnish researchers from the University of Helsinki showed that blocking NOS blocked "recovery sleep induction." On the other hand, boosting NO increased recovery sleep.

They also found that blocking iNOS decreased the "deep sleep" (non-REM sleep) phase of recovery sleep, while blocking nNOS decreased REM recovery sleep. They also found that increasing iNOS "evoked an increase in sleep that closely resembled recovery sleep."

Their conclusion: "NO is necessary and sufficient for the induction of recovery sleep," they wrote in the *European Journal of Neuroscience*.

Chronic Kidney Disease: The Role of NO

The kidneys filter and clean the blood, maintain the body's acid-alkaline balance, manufacture hormones that regulate blood pressure, and produce a form of vitamin D that strengthens the bones—in other words, they're absolutely essential to health.

But a lot of us *don't* have normal kidneys: chronic kidney disease (CKD) is a little-known epidemic that is damaging and destroying the kidneys of more than 26 million Americans. The cause of most cases of CKD: high blood pressure or type 2 diabetes.

NO can help protect your kidneys.

In the journal *Acta Physiologica*, a team of Australian researchers note that NO "has numerous important functions" in the kidney, including:

- regulating blood flow to the kidney.
- maintaining blood supply to the medulla, the inner region of the kidney.
- regulating the excretion of sodium.
- regulating the rate at which the kidney filters blood.

Writing in the journal *Clinica Chimica Acta*, a team of Polish researchers noted that chronic kidney disease is "invariably associated" with endothelial cell damage and low levels of NO.

In a study in the journal *Diabetes*, Italian researchers found that people with diabetics and kidney disease (diabetic nephropathy) synthesized NO at rates 37 percent lower than healthy people.

They also found the ability of the hormone insulin to stimulate the production of NO (one of its jobs) was *seven times* lower in people with diabetes and kidney disease.

And there's more evidence of the link between CKD and NO.

ADMA: The NO-blocking compound that damages kidneys

In an animal experiment, French researchers took a close look at the compound ADMA (asymmetric dimethylarginine), which *blocks* eNOS, the enzyme that sparks the production of NO in the endothelium. They found that administering ADMA created high blood pressure, damaged cells in the kidney, and led to scarring (fibrosis) of kidney cells.

Endothelial dysfunction—the result of too little NO—could "contribute to chronic kidney disease progression," concluded the researchers in the *Journal of Pathology*.

ADMA levels predict poor kidney function

In a study in the journal *Nephrology Dialysis Transplantation*, Polish researchers noted that heart disease and CKD are what they called *bidirectional*: kidney problems increase the risk of heart disease; heart disease speeds up loss of kidney function.

In their study of 80 men with diabetes who had undergone a surgical procedure to widen their arteries (angiography), they found that the best (and only) biochemical predictor of declining kidney function was rising levels of blood ADMA.

"Elevated ADMA may contribute to accelerated renal [kidney] function decline," they concluded. "This could result from the impairment of . . . endothelial renewal in the kidney, an NO-dependent process."

And in a scientific paper in the *Journal of Nephrology*, German researchers summed up the situation this way: "In patients with chronic kidney disease (CKD), ongoing endothelial damage in the capillary system [the tiniest blood vessels] of the renal [kidney] medulla . . . are thought to be central processes toward progressive kidney damage. In this respect, reduced nitric oxide synthesis by endothelial cells due to accumulation of endogenous inhibitors of the nitric oxide synthase such as asymmetric dimethylarginine (ADMA) has been accused of accelerating progression."

ADMA is guilty as charged—and there's a lot of work to formulate, test, and market a drug to block the formation of ADMA.

In the meantime, if you have kidney-damaging diabetes or high blood pressure, finding ways to boost your levels of NO may be one of the best strategies to keep your kidneys healthy or slow the progression of CKD.

Depression: Feeling Low on Low NO

Depression is a *very* common problem: doctors write about 230 million prescriptions for antidepressants every year. NO may help those drugs work.

Antidepressants are pro-NO

In a study of 70 people, those who were depressed had "significantly lower" levels of NO than those who weren't, reported Japanese researchers. And when the researchers treated the depressed people with an antidepressant, NO levels "significantly increased" in four weeks.

"Decreased blood levels of NO might be partially associated with the pathophysiology [development] of depression," concluded the researchers in the journal *Progress in Neuro-Psychopharmacology and Biological Psychiatry*.

In a similar study from researchers in the Department of Psychiatry at the University of Alberta in Canada, blood levels of NO were "significantly lower" in people with depression compared to people who weren't depressed, and treatment with an antidepressant increased NO levels.

Memory Loss: Don't Forget NO!

Can't remember where you put your keys? You may have lost your NO, too.

"There is an impressive amount of evidence suggesting the involvement of NO in . . . learning and memory," wrote a team of Iranian researchers in the journal *Behavioural Brain Research*.

NO is a must for good memory

In their animal study, the researchers found that blocking the production of NO hurt both short- and long-term memory, and that giving the animals NO-boosting L-arginine countered memory problems.

An animal study by Israeli researchers, in the *Journal of Neuroscience*, showed that NO is a must for forming short-term, intermediate-term, and long-term memories.

And in another animal study, Argentine researchers found that NO is required for the storage and retrieval of memory. Their findings were in the journal *Neurobiology of Learning and Memory*.

Osteoporosis: NO for Strong Bones

One out of every two women over 50 ends up with a broken bone because of *osteoporosis*—eroded and weakened bones. NO might play a role in preventing the problem.

Nitric oxide is "an important regulator of bone remodeling"—the creation of new bone, observed Dutch researchers in a study in the *Journal of Dental Research.*

And writing in the *Journal of Bone and Mineral Research*, UK researchers observed that any "mechanical strain" on the bone—for example, the type produced by weight-bearing exercise such as walking—generates more NO from bone cells called osteocytes.

Stopping bone loss with NO

NO can stop bone destruction by cells called *osteoclasts* and stimulate bone-building by cells called *osteoblasts*, observed Finnish researchers, in the medical journal *Bone.*

In an animal study, the researchers found that the NO-increasing drug nitroglycerin prevented bone loss.

"Nitrates [which generate NO] may be beneficial in conditions where bone turnover is compromised, such as in osteoporosis," concluded the researchers.

Overweight: Increased NO Is Why
Weight Loss Surgery Helps Your Heart

When you're carrying extra pounds, the fat weighs on your endothelium, cutting the production of NO and increasing your risk of heart disease. If you have weight loss surgery (bariatric surgery) and lose weight, your risk of heart disease is also lower—once again, because of NO.

A team of Polish researchers measured blood NO levels six months after successful weight loss surgery in 25 extremely obese people—and found their NO levels were 40 percent higher than before the surgery. The formerly obese patients also had drops in blood pressure, blood fats, and insulin levels.

"The increase of serum [blood] NO concentration contributes to diverse beneficial effects of weight loss after bariatric surgery," concluded the researchers in the journal *Obesity Surgery.*

Preeclampsia of Pregnancy: Baby Yourself with NO

This condition of sudden high blood pressure and excess protein in the urine strikes an estimated 5 to 8 percent of pregnant women after 20 weeks of pregnancy. Along with distressing symptoms such as swelling, headaches, and vision changes, preeclampsia can threaten the life of mother and baby: worldwide, it kills 76 thousand mothers and 500 thousand babies every year.

Preeclamptics have low NO

Brazilian researchers studied 94 pregnant women—47 healthy, 47 preeclamptic—and found those with preeclampsia had higher levels of ADMA and lower levels of nitrite, a NO precursor.

"These results may have important implications for studies on NO biology and therapeutic approaches of preeclampsia," concluded the researchers in the journal *Clinica Chimica Acta*. In other words, boosting NO may protect against high blood pressure and preeclampsia in pregnant women.

In a similar study, Chinese researchers measured blood levels of NO in women with preeclampsia—and found a "highly significant decrease" compared to healthy pregnant women.

Boosting NO levels "may represent a novel therapy for the treatment of preeclampsia," the researchers concluded in the journal *Archives of Gynecology and Obstetrics*.

Premature Babies: Protecting Lungs with NO

Tiny premature babies (less than three pounds) on respirators can develop *bronchopulmonary dysplasia* (BPD), a chronic lung disease with scarring and inflammation. Some treatments to prevent the condition can cause brain damage.

Researchers at Case Western Reserve University conducted a study involving 477 premature infants on respirators, following them until they were two years old. They found that treating the preemies with inhaled NO improved their chances of surviving without BPD and without neurological damage.

Inhaled NO is also the main therapy for treating newborns with a condition called pulmonary hypertension.

Schizophrenia: Preventing Drug Side Effects

A side effect of the drugs used to treat schizophrenia is *tardive dyskinesia* (TD): uncontrollable facial movements.

In an animal study by Indian researchers, NO-increasing compounds such as L-arginine blocked experimentally induced TD.

The study indicated "the potential of NO donors as a possible therapeutic option" in TD, concluded the researchers in the journal *Pharmacology Biochemistry and Behavior.*

Sickle Cell Anemia: Can NO Help?

This inherited and incurable disease warps the round shape of oxygen-carrying red blood cells into rigid, sticky "sickles"—curved slices of cells, like crescent moons. The misshapen cells snag and stall in the bloodstream, choking the flow of blood and oxygen and producing the disease's main symptoms: intense pain and damage to multiple organs.

"Endothelial dysfunction and impaired nitric oxide bioavailability have been implicated in the pathogenesis [disease progression] of sickle cell anemia," wrote researchers from the Boston University School of Medicine in a study in the *Journal of Cellular Physiology.* In particular, they noted, this reduced bioavailability of NO can lead to pulmonary hypertension (high blood pressure in the arteries that supply the lungs), which occurs in 30 to 40 percent of people with sickle cell anemia.

And in a paper in the journal *Free Radical Biology and Medicine* reviewing the links between sickle cell anemia and NO, researchers from the National Institutes of Health conclude that the "bioinactivation of NO" in the disease causes tighter blood vessels, less blood flow, more blood clotting, and end-organ injury.

One of the obvious keys to more effective treatment of the disease: "increase NO bioavailability," wrote the researchers.

Skin Diseases: Less Sun Damage with NO?

"It has become clear that this extraordinary molecular messenger [NO] plays a vital role in the skin, orchestrating normal regulatory processes," noted a team of French researchers in the medical journal *Nitric Oxide*.

The researchers listed the many roles NO performs in the skin, including:

- Keratinocytes, the main cells in the epidermis, the outer layer of skin, "express" iNOS, one the three nitric oxide synthase enzymes that trigger the production of NO. (And, they added, "under certain conditions virtually all skin cells appear to be capable of expressing" iNOS.)
- NO plays a role in the maintenance of the "barrier function"—the all-important role of the skin in keeping out unwanted germs and toxins.
- NO may help protect keratinocytes from damage and death from the sun's UV radiation.
- When the skin is wounded, NO helps guide the healing process, leading immune cells to the wound site.

"NO production," they concluded, seems "to play an important part in organizing the skin's unique adaptability and function."

Stomach Ulcers: NO for Prevention and Healing

Polish researchers found that pretreatment with NO-boosting compounds could prevent stomach ulcers in stressed rats. The findings were in the *Journal of Physiology and Pharmacology*.

And an animal study by Canadian researchers—published in the *American Journal of Physiology: Gastrointestinal and Liver Physiology*—found that NO production was key in the healing of stomach ulcers.

Stress: The Soothing Power of NO

Chronic stress causes or complicates nearly every disease, from heartburn to heart attacks. "Ninety percent of all health problems are stress-related," we were told by Kathleen Hall, PhD, director of the Stress Institute in Atlanta and author of *A Life in Balance*.

In an animal study, Indian researchers stressed laboratory animals by immobilizing them for six hours. Treating a group of those animals with antidepressants "significantly reversed immobilized stress-induced behaviors"—and treating the animals with those antidepressants *and* a NO-boosting compound calmed the stress-induced behaviors even more.

The study highlights "the involvement of NO mechanism in the protective effect against" stress, concluded the researchers in the journal *Neuroscience Letters*.

Conclusion

In these two chapters of Part I, we hope that we've helped you see that NO is indeed a miracle molecule, capable of protecting and restoring your health in many different ways.

Next, in Part II, we'll discuss the many different ways you can *boost* NO: with exercise; with a diet that emphasizes vegetables and NO-increasing plant compounds; with a NO-raising nutritional supplement; and with everyday lifestyle changes, such as getting more sleep and taking a warm bath.

• PART TWO •

Say Yes to NO

THREE

NOtrition:
NO-Boosting Foods
and Supplements

Go for the Leafy Greens

There's a scientific revolution in progress—and it's happening on your plate.

Let's look at a little history.

In 1998, scientists won the Nobel Prize for discovering that the gas nitric oxide—NO—was a signaling molecule in the lining of arteries (endothelium) and a *must* factor in the prevention of high blood pressure, heart disease, and stroke.

Next, those same Nobel-winning scientists (along with others) set out to discover practical ways to *boost* NO in the body. The main strategy they settled on: taking the supplement L-arginine, an amino acid that triggers eNOS (the enzyme endothelial nitric oxide synthase) to make NO.

The strategy seemed logical and straightforward—and likely to be effective. But although some studies have been positive about the use of L-arginine in heart disease, it didn't work nearly as well as hoped, especially in people 40 and older.

One study (which we'll describe in detail later in this chapter) showed that people who have had a heart attack *don't* benefit from supplemental L-arginine—and, in fact, shouldn't take it! Another study showed that people with peripheral arterial disease (clogged arteries in the legs) do *worse* when taking L-arginine over the long-term. ("No benefit and possible harm," was the conclusion about L-arginine reached by the researchers who conducted the study.)

But does that mean that nutritional strategies—eating foods and taking dietary supplements—*can't* boost NO?

To the contrary.

In the past decade, there's been a breakthrough in our scientific understanding of how nutrition impacts NO—a breakthrough with huge implications for your health.

We now know that there are pathways in the body that are *not* dependent on L-arginine to generate NO. Pathways that can convert foods rich in nitrate and nitrite (foods you can find in the produce section of your local supermarket, such as spinach, broccoli, and beets) into circulation-increasing, heart-protecting NO.

Let's look at the details of this fascinating scientific story—and the newest understanding of how you can use everyday foods and a nitrate-rich supplement to increase the level of NO in your body.

Is NO the Secret of Healthy Diets?

There is a lot of research pointing to the heart-protecting effect of a diet rich in vegetables and fruits. And scientists have tried to pinpoint just what it is about those foods that does the trick.

Is it the vitamins? The minerals? The fiber? The flavonols (a type of plant compound, or polyphenol), such as the resveratrol in grapes, the lutein in tomatoes, or the anthocyanins in blueberries?

As a strategy to isolate the individual heart-protecting nutrients in vegetables and fruits, studies have been conducted on nutritional supplements, such as the beta-carotene in vegetables, the vitamin C in fruits, or the vitamin E in vegetable oils. But more often than not, those studies failed to show any benefit in lowering the risk of heart attack, stroke, and other cardiovascular diseases. In fact, some research indicates that taking high doses of a single nutrient such as beta-carotene or vitamin E may *increase* the risk of disease!

The Mediterranean diet

Another way that scientists investigate the healing power of vegetables and fruits is by looking at the health effects of regional diets that feature plenty of produce.

One such diet, of course, is the much-touted Mediterranean diet, with its emphasis on vegetables, fruits, fish (rather than red meat), beans, whole grains, red wine, and monounsaturated olive oil as the main source of fat (rather than saturated fat from meat and dairy products).

For example, researchers from the Alpert Medical School of Brown University recently conducted a six-year diet and health study of more than 13 thousand people. Their results, in the journal *Atherosclerosis*, showed that those who adhered to a Mediterranean-style diet had:

- lower total cholesterol (a risk factor for heart disease).
- lower levels of C-reactive protein (a biomarker for chronic inflammation, which causes and complicates CVD).
- lower levels of hemoglobin A1c (a sign of better long-term blood sugar control; high blood sugar levels damage arteries).
- lower fibrinogen (a protein that increases the likelihood of the blood clots that cause most heart attacks and strokes).
- higher HDL cholesterol (which carries artery-clogging LDL cholesterol away from the heart).
- lower triglycerides (a blood fat that can hurt the heart in high levels).
- lower homocysteine (a biochemical linked to heart disease).

In another recent study on the Mediterranean diet and heart health, researchers from the Institute of Nutraceuticals and Functional Foods at Laval University in Canada studied 26 men who went on the Mediterranean diet for five weeks. The diet decreased total cholesterol by 7 percent and LDL by 9 percent, and (when the men also lost weight, a common "side effect" of eating Mediterranean-style) decreased blood pressure by up to 8 percent and triglycerides by 18 percent.

And in a five-year study of nearly 14 thousand people who didn't have cardiovascular disease at the beginning of the study, Spanish researchers found that those with the greatest adherence to a Mediterranean diet had a 59 percent lower risk of developing cardiovascular disease (CVD) or having heart attacks or strokes.

"There is an inverse association between adherence to the Mediterranean diet and the incidence of fatal and nonfatal CVD in initially healthy middle-aged adults," concluded the researchers in the journal *Nutrition, Metabolism and Cardiovascular Disease*.

But what *exactly* about the Mediterranean diet is so healthful for the heart and the entire body? Is it the olive oil, as many believe? Is it the red wine, as others say? Is it the *absence* of disease-causing factors, such as saturated fat?

That's the question that was asked by researchers from the University of Athens and the Harvard School of Public Health. In a nine-year study, they analyzed the diets of 23 thousand people, trying to find a link between specific factors of the Mediterranean diet and lower death rates from any cause, including heart disease.

The winner?

In vino veritas: wine had the greatest effect, linked to a 24 percent lower death rate. The silver medal went to what people *weren't* eating: a low intake of meat was linked to a 17 percent lower death rate.

But what *food* had the most effect on longevity? Not olive oil. Not fish or seafood. Not beans. Not nuts and seeds. Not even fruits.

No, it was *vegetables*—which lowered the death rate by 16 percent, much more than the foods just mentioned.

Green leafy vegetables

Stella Metsovas, CN, is a nutritionist in Laguna Beach, California, and both her parents are from Greece. She told us that the vegetable that's most prominent in the traditional Mediterranean diet of Crete (the "poster isle" of the Mediterranean diet) is *horta*, or boiled wild greens.

"In Crete, literally half the dietary intake is from horta," she said. (Comparable greens in the US would be dandelion greens, mustard greens, collards, and beet greens.)

Well (and this is a *very* important point), dark leafy greens are among the foods richest in nitrate and nitrite, two dietary compounds that create NO in the body. In fact, a study shows that the typical Mediterranean diet—rich in leafy greens—may contain up to *20 times* more nitrate and nitrite than a typical Western diet.

And when you take a close look at some of the scientific research on the health-promoting power of vegetables, you find that leafy green vegetables are often the standouts.

Leafy greens lower heart disease risk by 18 percent. In an analysis of diet and heart disease among more than 100 thousand people, Portuguese researchers found that those who regularly ate nitrate-rich green leafy vegetables had an 18 percent lower risk of developing CVD. The findings were in the journal *Public Health Nutrition.*

And the risk of stroke by 21 percent. In a study by researchers from the Harvard School of Public Health of more than 100 thousand people, those who ate the most leafy green vegetables had a 21 percent lower risk of having a stroke compared to those who ate the least. Additionally, those who ate the most nitrate-rich cruciferous vegetables (such as broccoli, cauliflower, and cabbage) had a 32 percent lower risk. The results were in the *Journal of the American Medical Association.*

Leafy greens are the standout. Another study from Harvard School of Public Health, in the *Annals of Internal Medicine*, produced similar results. Researchers analyzed diet and health data from more than 126 thousand people and found that those with the highest intake of vegetables and fruits had a 20 percent lower risk of heart disease—and that nitrate-rich green leafy vegetables (along with vitamin C–rich fruits and vegetables) "contributed most to the . . . protective effect of total fruit and vegetable intake." In fact, just having *one more serving a day* of green leafy vegetables decreased risk by 23 percent!

The DASH diet

There's another diet in which increased vegetable and fruit intake plays a prominent role in the prevention of cardiovascular disease: the Dietary Approaches to Stop Hypertension (DASH) diet, specifically designed to lower high blood pressure.

The diet "prescribes" 8 to 10 servings of vegetables and fruits a day, along with low-fat dairy products—and scientific findings show that it's just as effective as medication in lowering high blood pressure. In a recent study by researchers from the Johns Hopkins University School of Medicine, the DASH diet reduced the 10-year risk of heart disease by 18 percent.

"In addition to reducing blood pressure, the DASH diet should substantially reduce the risk of coronary heart disease," the researchers concluded in the journal *Circulation: Cardiovascular Quality and Outcomes*.

How does the DASH diet work? Researchers have different theories.

Maybe it's the high levels of the mineral calcium, which is known to help relax arteries and is linked to protection from heart disease. Maybe it's the mineral potassium, also linked to lower blood pressure. Maybe it's the polyphenols in the diet, including the flavonols. Or the fiber. Or the fact that the diet restricts pressure-boosting salt and artery-clogging red meat.

But we have a *different* idea about why the DASH diet (and the Mediterranean diet) work to lower blood pressure and the risk of heart disease and stroke.

We think those diets work because of their high level of NO-boosting nitrate and nitrite.

Nitrate and Nitrite: The Secret, Heart-Saving Ingredients in Vegetable-Rich Diets

Here's a one-sentence summary of why we think the Mediterranean diet and the DASH diet are healthy for hearts:

The *nitrate* in the vegetables turns into *nitrite* and *nitric oxide* (NO)— and these compounds expand arteries (vasodilation), decrease blood pressure, and protect the heart from a heart attack and the brain from a stroke.

Now let's look in depth at the new scientific discoveries that are revealing how and why dietary nitrate and nitrite is the *best* way to boost NO.

As we've discussed previously (but never tire of repeating), the healthy functioning of your circulatory system demands NO and the ability of blood vessels to respond to the signal from NO to relax and expand.

The production of NO depends on the enzyme eNOS (endothelial

DASH-ed Hopes for High NO

Dr. Bryan's laboratory has tested a wide variety of foods for their nitrate and nitrite content—and found that *even if* you follow the DASH diet religiously, eating 8 to 10 servings of fruits and/or vegetables a day, you might not achieve a very high level of NO intake.

A day of eating fruits and vegetables on a DASH diet that supplies a lot of nitrate (1,222 mg) and nitrite (0.351 mg) looks like this:

1 cup raw spinach	¼ cup raisins
½ cup cooked collard greens	1 medium orange
½ cup vegetable juice	½ cup pomegranate juice
1 medium banana	

A day of eating fruits and vegetables on a DASH that doesn't supply a lot of nitrate (174 mg) and nitrite (0.41 mg) looks like this:

1 cup raw leaf lettuce	¼ cup raisins
½ cup broccoli	½ cup canned fruit juice cocktail
½ cup vegetable juice	½ cup orange juice
1 medium apple	

Bottom line: you can end up with *seven times* less NO-producing nitrate on the same diet! The solution to this problem?

If you're on the DASH diet:

1. Emphasize foods high on the NO Index (which we'll discuss in a moment).
2. Consider an NO-boosting dietary supplement (also discussed below).
3. Follow the NO-boosting exercise and lifestyle recommendations in Chapters 4 and 5.

nitric oxide synthase) and two other similar enzymes (nNOS and iNOS), which synthesize NO from L-arginine and oxygen.

With NO on board, the vessels expand (vasodilation), blood pressure is regulated, the lining of the endothelium is resistant to invasion by sticky plaque-creating immune factors, and there's less of a tendency for tiny components in the blood to form an artery-plugging blood clot (platelet aggregation).

Two more ways to create NO

But the production of NO isn't *only* dependent on eNOS and the presence of L-arginine. The body has a backup. In fact, there are *several* additional systems that "reduce" nitrate to nitrite, so that nitrite can turn into NO. (*Reduce* is a technical term used in chemistry for a process that turns one chemical compound into another.)

The first system is in your digestive tract: friendly bacteria on the tongue reduce some of the nitrate in saliva into nitrite. (The amount of nitrate and nitrite in saliva depends almost entirely on the amount of nitrate in *food*.) When you swallow that nitrite, it either produces NO or is absorbed in the digestive tract and sent throughout the body.

When you swallow nitrate, about 25 percent is absorbed in the small intestine and shunted back to your salivary glands—where bacteria *again* reduce the nitrate to nitrite.

This is one of the body's recycling systems: a clever way to *continuously* produce nitrite, so it's always available to convert into NO.

The second system (yet another recent scientific discovery shaking up the understanding of how NO works): NO creation occurs in the body's tissues. In fact, scientists in Sweden at the famous Karolinska Institute have shown that several enzymes and proteins—not just bacteria on the tongue and in the gut—can reduce nitrate to NO. Even the body's mitochondria—the tiny energy factories in every cell—have been shown to possess "nitrate reductase activity."

All in all, scientists are now estimating that the nitrate and nitrite in the diet may supply *50 percent* of the body's NO!

In a recent scientific paper published in the *American Journal of Clinical Nutrition*, Dr. Bryan and several colleagues called these "backup" systems for the formation of NO "elegant physiologically redundant mechanisms . . . to ensure an abundant supply of nitric oxide for the myriad of processes that require them."

Let's summarize the scientific info we just presented by listing the many ways you can create and re-create NO.

1. Dietary nitrate enters the body by mouth and is reduced to nitrite, which the body can convert to NO in the stomach or tissues.
2. Dietary nitrite enters the body by mouth and is reduced to NO.
3. L-arginine combines with oxygen to create NO, sparked by the nitric oxide synthase (NOS) enzymes.
4. NO is oxidized *back* to nitrite or other so-called nitrogen oxides (chemically symbolized by NOx), which are then recycled to the saliva or tissues and re-reduced to NO.

In other words, the body doesn't just have *one* way to create NO. Because NO is so important, it has *many* ways, including forming NO from nitrate and nitrite.

But those statements are about science. What does it mean for *you* that the body can reduce nitrate to nitrite, and nitrite to NO?

It means you can use *dietary* means—foods rich in nitrate and nitrite, or a supplement that supplies nitrate and nitrite—to strengthen and regenerate your cardiovascular system.

Let's explore the best ways to do just that.

Putting more greens in your diet

What's the right amount of leafy greens for health?

"Everyone should consume five or more servings of vegetables a day," said Ann Kulze, MD, founder and CEO of Just Wellness in Charleston, South Carolina, and author of *Dr. Ann's 10-Step Diet.*

"A serving is a half-cup raw or cooked of any vegetables *except* dark leafy greens," she told us. "For dark leafy greens, such as spinach, one serving is one cup uncooked."

To get advice on *how* to include more of those leafy green vegetables in the diet, we talked with Steven Pratt, MD, author of the best-selling book *SuperFoods Rx*, and a physician at the Scripps Memorial Hospital in La Jolla, California.

Here are his tips for buying and eating plenty of leafy greens:

Is Nitrate the Answer?

That's the question an international team of scientists from the world-famous Karolinska Institute in Sweden and from Boston University School of Medicine asked themselves while wondering *why* vegetables protect the heart from disease.

In their scientific paper in the medical journal *Nitric Oxide*—"Cardioprotective effects of vegetables: Is nitrate the answer?"—the researchers offer this perspective:

1. Eating a diet rich in vegetables lowers blood pressure almost as much as treatment with a standard pressure-lowering drug.
2. The high content of nitrate in certain vegetables, and its conversion to nitrite and NO, is the real reason why vegetables are cardioprotective.
3. In fact, this pathway of NO generation works *better* than the L-arginine pathway, which "malfunctions" in people with heart disease.
4. Vegetarians (who have low rates of heart disease) consume about 10 times more nitrate than nonvegetarians, as do people who eat

Shopping. "Look for fresh-looking, fresh-smelling greens," he said. "Avoid any that are yellowed, browned, slimy, or wilting."

Dr. Pratt also recommends buying prewashed baby spinach. "They're perhaps the quickest and easiest of all leafy green vegetables, taking just a minute or two to prepare," he told us. "Just heat up, add a squeeze of lemon juice and a drizzle of extra-virgin olive oil, and you've got a side dish."

He urges a bit of caution, however, when buying bagged greens. "Check for expiration dates. And check for dark soggy leaves, which means the greens are past their prime."

Refrigeration. Once you bring the greens home, refrigerate them—but with one extra step. "Keep them moist but not wet," said Dr. Pratt. "Roll them lightly in damp paper towels and store the bundle in a plastic bag, with holes punched in it so the humidity doesn't promote spoilage."

a Mediterranean-style diet, also shown to protect against heart disease.

5. The task for scientists is to find the *optimal level* of nitrate and nitrite intake for cardioprotection.

Their conclusions:

6. "...the protective effect of certain vegetables on the cardiovascular system is related to their high content of nitrate."
7. "The mechanism involves reduction of dietary nitrate to nitrite [and] nitric oxide."
8. "A continuous intake of nitrate-containing food such as green leafy vegetables may ensure that tissue levels of NO...are maintained..."
9. "If proven true, these considerations could have a profound impact on our view of the role of diet...in the...prevention of cardiovascular disease."

They took the words right out of our mouths!

Preparation. Don't wash the greens until right before you use them, he advised.

Maximize at meals. To maximize your intake of spinach, he recommends making extra hot, steamed spinach and having it as a cold side dish for lunch, with a drizzle of soy dressing or lemon juice. You can also add spinach (and other greens) to salads regularly, or to soups and casseroles. You can "dress up" steamed or sautéed greens with a sprinkle of toasted sesame seeds or pine nuts, he told us. And you can use spinach and other dark leafy greens instead of lettuce on sandwiches.

NO-boosting tips

Here are some additional dietary tips to boost NO.

Add lemon. Putting some lemon—rich in vitamin C—on cooked greens or salads helps increase the conversion of nitrate and nitrite to NO.

The Best Part

Different *parts* of vegetables are higher in nitrate than others. From the most to the least, the order is:

1. Stalk of the leaf (the petiole, which attaches the leaf to the plant)
2. Leaf
3. Stem (the part of the plant that supports the leaves and/or flowers)
4. Root
5. Flower
6. Bulb
7. Fruit
8. Seed

Enjoy watermelon. It's high in citrulline—an amino acid that helps your body make NO.

Have an NO smoothie. Blend a combination of vegetables: 1 zucchini, 1 stalk of celery, 2 pieces of kale, a squirt of lemon juice, your favorite seasoning, plus tomato juice or water to taste.

Trade in soda for fruit juice or tea. As we'll discuss in a moment, pomegranate juice, apple juice, or green or black tea are terrific ways to help your body boost NO.

Drink plenty of water. As we discuss in Chapter 5, staying hydrated helps you make more NO.

The Power of Polyphenols

Polyphenols—antioxidant plant compounds—are the celebrities of the nutritional world.

There's *resveratrol*, the polyphenol in red wine that some scientists think could be a key to superlongevity.

There's *EGCG* (epigallocatechin gallate), the polyphenol in green and black tea that thousands of scientific studies show may help protect you against (don't hold your breath while reading the rest of this sentence): aging, allergies, Alzheimer's disease, bladder cancer, breast cancer, cervical cancer, cholesterol problems, colon cancer, diabetes, flu, fungal infections, heart attack, immune weakness, leukemia, Lou Gehrig's disease, lung cancer, the metabolic syndrome, pancreatic cancer, prostate cancer, skin cancer, stomach cancer, stroke, ulcers, and weight gain. (We told you it was a long list, but that's a powerful polyphenol for you.)

There are the *anthocyanins*, the polyphenols in blueberries that recent research shows can slow memory loss in 70-year-olds.

Then there are polyphenol-rich foods much touted for their heart-protecting power, such as red wine and chocolate.

But as much press as polyphenols receive, they have an ability that's rarely discussed in the media: their ability to boost NO.

Let's look at that ability food by food.

Apples

Italian researchers found that two polyphenols in an apple extract increased NO release in the saliva. "Some apple polyphenols . . . promote NO bio-availability at the gastric [stomach] level, a previously unappreciated function," concluded the researchers in the journal *Free Radical Biology and Medicine*.

Red wine

As you probably know, moderate intake of alcohol (two drinks a day for men, and one drink a day for women) has been linked to a healthier heart—and even to longevity. Studies link moderate drinking to:

- 42 percent lower risk of heart attack or death from heart disease.
- 32 percent lower risk of heart attack if you have high blood pressure.
- 34 percent lower risk of congestive heart failure.
- 23 percent lower risk of stroke.

Some researchers have focused on the unique power of red wine to convey those benefits, and scientists have focused on several factors: the ethanol, the resveratrol, and the tannins (polyphenols called *anthocyanins*). But could NO have something to do with it, too? Yes, say scientific studies.

Compounds in red wine increase NO. Portuguese researchers found that red wine—the wine itself; the anthocyanins; and catechol, another polyphenol—all promoted the production of NO when mixed with nitrite, in the test tube and in the bodies of healthy volunteers. "The reduction of nitrite may reveal previously unrecognized physiologic [physical] effects of red wine in connection with NO bioactivity," they concluded in *Free Radical Biology and Medicine.*

Wine-produced NO relaxes muscles. A few years later, the same team of researchers conducted an animal study showing that NO produced via red wine relaxed the wall of the stomach. "The results establish a link between the consumption of nitrite and dietary reductants (e.g. wine polyphenols) and stomach muscle relaxation via the local chemical generation of NO," concluded the researchers in the journal *Nitric Oxide.*

One more reason a little red wine with a meal is probably very good for you!

Pomegranate juice

Recent research on the healing power of pomegranate juice—rich in polyphenols—has been remarkable.

In one study, conducted by doctors from the Preventive Medicine Research Institute in Sausalito, California, and the University of California, people with severe heart disease who drank eight ounces of pomegranate juice a day for three months had a 17 percent increase in blood flow to the heart—compared to a similar group who didn't drink the juice and had an 18 percent decrease. The pomegranate-drinkers also had a 50 percent decrease in angina. In other research, pomegranate juice has helped stop the artery-clogging oxidation of LDL cholesterol and reversed arterial plaque by 30 percent.

Why does it work?

"Pomegranate juice contains powerful antioxidants such as polyphenols, tannins, and anthocyanins," Dr. Ornish told us.

But could pomegranate juice also influence NO production? Studies show the answer is yes.

Pomegranate increases NO in arterial cells. In a test tube and animal study by Italian researchers in the *Proceedings of the National Academy of Sciences*, a pomegranate concentrate increased the production of eNOS in endothelial cells that had been damaged by reduced blood flow. (The artery narrows; the blood flow turns from a calm and steady current into artery-battering rapids; the resulting injury is called "shear stress"—and shear stress decreases the production of eNOS.)

Pomegranate stops NO destruction. A year later, another team of scientists, at the David Geffen School of Medicine at UCLA, found that pomegranate juice protected NO from oxidative destruction, preserving it in the body.

A few months after that, the Italian scientists published research showing that pomegranate juice reverses the limited production of eNOS caused by high levels of oxidized LDL.

"Our data suggest that pomegranate juice can exert beneficial effects on the [development] of clinical vascular complications, coronary heart disease, and atherogenesis in humans by enhancing the eNOS bioactivity," they concluded in the journal *Nitric Oxide*.

Pomegranate restores lowered NO. Finally (at least for now), the Italian researchers showed that pomegranate fruit extract and pomegranate juice increased eNOS after it had been decreased by shear stress. They also noted that pomegranate increased nitrate levels. And that it had *no* effect on levels of L-arginine. (In other words, the polyphenols in pomegranate worked via the nitrate-nitrite-NO pathway, and *not* via the L-arginine pathway.) Those findings were in the journal *Cardiovascular Research*.

Cocoa

Many studies link cocoa-rich dark chocolate—packed with polyphenols—to heart health. In one of the most recent, researchers from the Karolinska Institute in Sweden and the Harvard School of Public Health surveyed more than 1,100 people who had lived through a heart attack, finding out how much chocolate they had eaten in the year before. Then they tracked their health for the next eight years. Compared to people who hadn't eaten any chocolate before their heart attack, eating chocolate reduced the risk of dying from heart disease by:

- 66 percent, eating chocolate twice or more a week.
- 44 percent, eating chocolate once a week.
- 27 percent, eating chocolate less than once a month.

In research in the *American Journal of Hypertension*, scientists analyzed data from 10 studies on flavonol-rich dark chocolate and blood pressure, and found eating dark chocolate lowered blood pressure by up to four points systolic (the upper reading) and six points diastolic (the lower reading).

When Canadian researchers analyzed diet and health data from more than 44 thousand people, they found that those who ate chocolate once a week were 22 percent less likely to have a stroke, compared to those who didn't eat chocolate.

Not surprisingly, researchers have also investigated the relationship of dark chocolate and NO, the key to the health of the cardiovascular system.

Dark chocolate improves endothelial function. Researchers at the Yale Prevention Research Center studied 45 people (average age 53), giving half the study participants a dark chocolate bar and the other half a cocoa-free bar. Later, half drank cocoa-rich dark chocolate and half didn't. After the study participants ate the bar and downed the drink, researchers measured their endothelial function: how much arteries widened and allowed blood flow.

The dark chocolate improved endothelial function 60 to 70 percent more than the non-cocoa products. And blood pressure decreased—a logical result of wider arteries. The findings were in the *American Journal of Clinical Nutrition*.

Dark chocolate beats heart disease because it increases NO. Researchers at Harvard Medical School asked 27 people to eat flavonol-rich dark chocolate for four days and then measured their vasodilation. Eating the dark chocolate "induced consistent and striking" vasodilation, observed the researchers. But when the participants were given an NO-blocking compound, the vasodilation stopped—proving the effects of the dark chocolate were from an increase in NO.

"In healthy humans, flavonol-rich cocoa induced vasodilation via activation of the nitric oxide system, providing a plausible mechanism for the protection that flavonol-rich foods induce against coronary events," wrote the researchers.

Dark chocolate lowers blood pressure—and boosts NO. In a study from Germany, researchers divided 44 people with either prehypertension (120/80 to 139/89 mm Hg) or Stage 1 hypertension (140/90 to 159/99 mm Hg) into two groups: every day, one group ate a small amount of dark chocolate (just a little bit bigger than a Hershey's Kiss) rich in polyphenols, while the other group ate the same amount of white chocolate (with no polyphenols). At the beginning and end of the study, the researchers measured blood pressure levels and also a biomarker of increased production of NO (S-nitrosoglutathione).

After 18 weeks, those in the dark chocolate group had an average drop in blood pressure of 2.9 systolic and 1.0 diastolic—low enough that the percentage of hypertensives in the group dropped from 86 to 68 percent. (In other words, their blood pressure was now low enough so that they were no longer officially diagnosed as hypertensive.)

There was also a "steady increase" in S-nitrosoglutathione.

"Inclusion of small amounts of polyphenol-rich dark chocolate as part of a usual diet efficiently reduced blood pressure and improved formation of vasodilative nitric oxide," concluded the researchers in the *Journal of the American Medical Association.*

More NO, less heart disease . . . and cancer . . . and diabetes. In a paper in *International Journal of Medical Sciences*, researchers from the University of Panama looked at the disease and death rates of the Kuna—a tribe of Indians living on an island off Panama who drink five cups a day of flavonol-rich dark chocolate as their main beverage (and incorporate cocoa into many other recipes), and "thus probably have the most flavonoid-rich diet of any population" in the world.

"Our hypothesis," wrote the researchers, "is that if the high flavonoid intake and consequent nitric oxide system activation were important, the results would be a reduction in the frequency of ischemic heart disease, stroke, diabetes mellitus, and cancer—all nitric oxide sensitive processes."

Well, the hypothesis was proven: when the researchers compared death and disease rates of the mainland population to that of the Kuna, they found rates of heart disease among the Kuna that were 89 percent lower, rates of cancer that were 94 percent lower, and rates of diabetes that were 73 percent lower.

"This comparatively lower risk among Kuna . . . from the most common causes of morbidity [ill health] and mortality [death] in much of the world, possibly reflect a very high flavonol intake and sustained nitric oxide synthesis activation," concluded the researchers.

NO-boosting dark chocolate even works in smokers. A team of German researchers studied 11 smokers—and found that drinking a flavonol-rich dark chocolate caused a "significant increase" of 28 percent in blood levels of NO.

"The circulating pool of bioactive NO and endothelium-dependent vasodilation is acutely increased in smokers following the oral ingestion of a flavonol-rich cocoa drink," concluded the researchers in the *Journal of the American College of Cardiology.* "This increase in circulating NO . . . may contribute to beneficial vascular health effects of flavonol-rich food."

So if you *must* smoke (and we hope you don't)—at least have a little bit of dark chocolate after you finish your cigarette!

Cocoa contributes nitrate and nitrite, too. In other research on the Kuna, scientists from Harvard Medical School note that they have a three-fold higher level of urinary nitrate/nitrite than the mainland population: in other words, cocoa is boosting NO not only by increasing levels of eNOS, but also by boosting blood levels of nitrate and nitrite.

How dark chocolate boosts NO. In a recent study, researchers in the Department of Medicine at the University of California–San Diego decided to conduct a test tube study on endothelial cells to figure out *how* dark chocolate worked to increase NO on the biochemical level. They found that treating the cells with epicatechin—a polyphenol in dark chocolate—activated a complex biochemical chain reaction in the membranes of endothelial cells that increased eNOS. The findings were in the journal *Hypertension.*

Black and green tea

Black and green tea start life the same way: as leaves on *Camellia sinensis,* an evergreen shrub that is cultivated as a bush on tea plantations. The leaves are picked and dried. In green tea, the drying (or fermentation) process is stopped by lightly steaming or pan-frying the leaves. In black tea, leaves are allowed to fully ferment. (Oolong tea is fermented longer than green tea but shorter than black.)

But black or green, the tea leaves contain goodly amounts of polyphenols called *catechins*—with the power to protect hearts.

Research shows the polyphenols in tea can:

- protect heart cells from oxidation.
- prevent oxidation of LDL cholesterol.
- reduce total cholesterol and LDL cholesterol.
- slow the growth of vascular smooth muscle cells, which narrow arteries.
- cut down on clot-causing platelet aggregation.

In a recent study in the *Journal of Epidemiology and Community Health*, Japanese researchers analyzed diet and health data from nearly 77 thousand people. They found women who drank the most green tea had a 42 percent lower risk of developing heart disease than those who drank the least. And in a seven-year study of more than 12 thousand people, in the *Annals of Epidemiology*, Japanese researchers found that those who drank the most tea were 24 percent less likely to die from heart disease than those who drank the least.

Could NO have anything to do with it? Definitely.

In a review of the topic, titled "Tea, Flavonoids, and Nitric-Oxide Mediated Vascular Reactivity" in the *Journal of Nutrition*, Italian researchers note that studies show:

Black tea triggers NOS activity and NO availability. Researchers at the Whitaker Cardiovascular Institute of the Boston University School of Medicine exposed artery endothelial cells to black tea polyphenols—and found the black tea "acutely enhances nitric oxide bioactivity." The findings were in the *Journal of Biological Chemistry*.

Green tea and black tea double NO-sparked blood flow. In a study in the *British Journal of Nutrition*, German researchers showed that drinking either green tea or black tea nearly doubled a NO-sparked widening of blood vessels and increase in blood flow.

"There is now consistent data indicating that tea and tea flavonoids

Don't Forget the Fish Oil

Fish oil—rich in the omega-3 essential fatty acids EPA (eicosapentae-noic acid) and DHA (docosahexaenoic acid)—is famous for healing hearts. More than three decades of research shows it can: slow the accumulation of artery-clogging plaque, helping to prevent a heart attack; prevent or treat arrhythmia (disordered heart rhythms that can cause sudden cardiac death); prevent or treat atrial fibrillation (a quiver in the upper chambers of the heart that increases the risk for blood clots and stroke); and strengthen the heart of someone with congestive heart disease.

There are many explanations for why eating fatty fish or taking a fish oil supplement is so effective. It lowers triglycerides, heart-hurting blood fats. It stabilizes plaque. It reduces inflammation, which fuels heart disease. It thins the blood. It tones the nervous system, which controls the heartbeat.

But—perhaps most importantly of all—scientific research shows that fish oil generates more NO.

Restoring endothelial health in kids with high blood fats.
Sometimes high cholesterol and/or high blood fats is inherited, a condition called *familial hypercholesterolemia* (FH) or *familial combined hyperlipidemia* (FCH). Twenty children and adolescents (ages 9 to 19) with FH or FCH took 1.2 grams of DHA or a placebo for six weeks; then they switched for six weeks, with the placebo group taking the DHA and vice versa. The researchers measured the degree of widening of the brachial artery in the upper arm—a standard way to test the health of the endothelium, which depends on the production of NO. (The test is called endothelium-dependent flow-mediated dilation, or FMD.)

"FMD increased significantly after DHA supplementation," concluded the researchers from the University of California–San Francisco, in the *International Journal of Clinical Pharmacology and Therapeutics*. "The endothelium may thus be a therapeutic target for DHA," they continued. "This is consistent with a hypothesis of increasing NO bioavailability, with the potential of preventing the progression of early coronary heart disease in high-risk children."

Fish oil works in adults, too. In a similar study, Australian researchers found that DHA supplements for six weeks improved the blood flow in the forearms of overweight men with high levels of blood fats. "Improvements in endothelium-independent mechanisms . . . may contribute to the . . . blood pressure–lowering effect observed with DHA . . . in humans," they concluded in the medical journal *Circulation*.

Fish oil boosts NO. And in a study conducted by researchers at the University of Kansas Medical Center, 29 people who took fish oil had an increase in their excretion of nitrate, a sign of increasing NO production. Fish oil "may stimulate systemic nitric oxide synthesis," which "suggests another mechanism whereby omega-3 fatty acids may be antiathero-genic," concluded the researchers in the *American Journal of Clinical Nutrition*.

What's the best way to get your fish oil?

If you have heart disease, the American Heart Association (AHA) recommends a daily dose of 1,000 mg (1 gram) of EPA and DHA. If you don't have heart disease, the AHA recommends you eat two oily fish meals a week, which is the equivalent of about 500 mg a day of EPA and DHA—the amount linked to the lowest risk of developing heart disease. (Oily fish include herring, mackerel, salmon, albacore tuna, sardines, and oysters.)

"However, very few people probably have two fish meals per week—the amount you need to average 500 mg a day," we were told by cardiologist and fish oil expert Carl L. Lavie, MD, medical director of Cardiac Rehabilitation and Prevention at the Ochsner Heart and Vascular Institute in New Orleans, Louisiana. "And the dosage that showed benefits in heart disease would require five fish meals a week," he continued. "So it may be far more practical to take a fish oil supplement."

Dr. Lavie recommends Lovaza, a prescription omega-3 supplement, which is guaranteed to deliver the specified amount of DHA and EPA. For over-the-counter brands, he prefers Nordic Naturals and GNC.

can enhance nitric oxide status and improve endothelial function, which may be at least partly responsible for benefits on cardiovascular health," concluded Australian researchers in a paper on tea flavonoids and cardiovascular health in the journal *Molecular Aspects of Medicine*.

Practical actions

What should you do on the basis of all this evidence about polyphenols and NO?

Well, an apple a day *does* keep the doctor away—particularly a cardiologist!

And don't just eat that apple. Enjoy all the unique polyphenol-rich foods that study after study shows are good for your heart—probably *because* they're helping to boost your levels of NO.

Enjoy a bite or two of dark chocolate a day, looking for a brand with a minimum of 75 percent cacao, the flavonol-rich ingredient. (Remember, you don't need much: the German researchers found an NO-boosting benefit with an amount of dark chocolate about one-third bigger than a Hershey's Kiss.)

Enjoy a cup or two a day of green or black tea.

Enjoy moderate intake of red wine. The classic Mediterranean style of drinking red wine for health: four ounces, once or twice a day, with meals, in a social and convivial atmosphere.

Enjoy a glass of pomegranate juice.

And then take the next step: pack your diet with foods high on the NO Index, which are rich in nitrate and nitrite *and* in the antioxidants (such as polyphenols) that provide biochemical protection for the nitrate-to-nitrite-to-NO pathway.

What's the NO Index? Read on.

The NO Index: A New (and Better) Way to Think about Foods

We'd like to orient you to the NO Index—recently created by Dr. Bryan and Dr. Zand—by first discussing another nutritional "index" that scientists have developed and the public has embraced: the Glycemic Index, a measurement of how quickly the body turns carbohydrates into blood sugar (glucose).

The Glycemic Index: a nutritional guide for diabetes

The Glycemic (GI) Index was invented by David Jenkins, PhD, a professor of nutrition at the University of Toronto, as a dietary tool for people with diabetes, who need to keep their high blood sugar levels under control. (Decades of high blood sugar damages the blood vessels of the circulatory system, from the river of an artery to the one-cell trickle of a capillary. This leads to the catastrophic complications of diabetes: heart disease, stroke, blindness, kidney failure, nerve damage, and hard-to-heal skin ulcers and subsequent toe, foot, and leg amputations. As you've read earlier, high NO levels can also help control diabetes.)

Fast-digesting carbohydrates high on the GI Index (such as white bread) push up blood sugar levels and are bad for people with diabetes. Slow-digesting carbohydrates low on the GI Index (such as beans) stabilize blood sugar levels and are good for people with diabetes.

And since modern nutritional science is showing that high blood sugar (and the high levels of the hormone insulin that the body pumps out to control it) are bad for just about every cell, organ, and system, the GI Index has become a tool not only for those with diabetes, but to help prevent and control overweight (rocketing and crashing high blood sugar levels addle the appetite), heart disease, the metabolic syndrome (a multiproblem condition featuring blood sugar problems, overweight, and high blood pressure), and even Alzheimer's.

The NO Index: a nutritional guide for heart disease and good health

Well, we think the NO Index of foods that we have created can do for heart disease what the Glycemic Index has done for diabetes. In fact, we think the NO Index can do more for all-around health than any other nutritional guideline, because maintaining high levels of NO is *the* all-important factor in maintaining good health, especially for people 40 and older.

We have calculated the NO Index using two factors.

1. The total amount of NO-creating nitrate and nitrite in a food.
2. The ORAC (oxygen radical absorption capacity) of a food—its amount of antioxidants.

Let's look at those factors one by one, and why they're important.

Nitrate and nitrite. As we explained earlier in this chapter, the body uses nitrate and nitrite in foods to generate and maintain NO levels—chemically speaking, the body "reduces" nitrate and nitrite to NO. That's why foods with high levels of nitrate and nitrite—such as dark leafy greens—are high on the NO Index.

Antioxidants. But it's not only important to *generate* NO. It's also important to *preserve* NO, so the body can use it. And then *regenerate* more NO from the body's breakdown of compounds called nitrogen dioxides. To do all that, you need *antioxidants*: compounds that stop oxidants (also called "radical oxygen species," or "free radicals") from reacting with NO. If you don't stop those oxidants, they'll not only wipe out NO, but also form potentially dangerous N-nitrosamine compounds.

Nutritional scientists use the ORAC scale to measure antioxidants because it shows actual antioxidant *activity*—the food's ability to limit and stop the type of oxidation reactions that dismantle NO.

As you'll see in the listing of NO Index foods below, the foods "high" on the NO Index are *vegetables*—they're loaded with nitrate and nitrite *and* with antioxidants. Vegetables also dominate the "medium" range of the index, with some fruits and grains added. A variety of foods are "low" in the NO Index. (We're not saying to avoid those "low" foods—many of which are healthy foods, such as sweet potatoes, onions, and cherries—but only to emphasize the "high" and "medium" foods.)

We want to emphasize that the NO Index is a very new tool, just entering into the realm of scientific and medical literature, and books such as this one. But we think over time it will prove itself to be a very successful invention, like the Glycemic Index.

Understanding a food's ranking on the NO Index will help explain many scientific findings about the health benefits of some foods (such as green leafy vegetables).

A diet emphasizing foods high on the NO Index may provide an even better diet for lowering high blood pressure than the DASH guidelines; in fact, eating foods high on the NO Index will provide a means to prevent the progression of existing heart disease.

The NO Index should become a way for primary care physicians to guide their patients with risk factors for heart disease (high blood pressure, high LDL cholesterol, low HDL cholesterol, etc.) in the daily production of more NO—a way that actually *works*, as compared to taking a nutritional supplement of L-arginine. (You can read more about L-arginine and heart disease in the section on supplements to boost NO.)

A diet loaded with foods high on the NO Index may be used to boost NO before open heart surgery or heart transplant surgery—improving the odds of a positive postsurgical outcome.

And since high levels of NO can protect you from a number of conditions other than heart disease, eating meals loaded with foods high on the NO Index will become a way to prevent diabetes or reverse the metabolic syndrome.

The possibilities for using the NO Index for health and healing are virtually endless. But they start right here!

On page 64, you'll find a preliminary listing of foods that are high, medium, and low on the NO Index—and we urge you to emphasize those high and medium foods! To make that as easy as possible, we've also provided 12 recipes that feature foods that are high and medium on the NO Index—and a three-day meal plan that suggests how those might be used for breakfasts, lunches, and dinners.

Our hope is to continually test more and more foods, adding them to the NO Index, and then to conduct clinical studies of the effectiveness of using the NO Index to lower high blood pressure and to control heart disease and other health problems. As you now know, using *foods* to boost NO is a new and largely uncharted advance in the science of health.

Welcome to the adventure!

The NO Index					
HIGH		**MEDIUM**		**LOW**	
Kale	6825	Coleslaw	84	String beans	9
Swiss chard	2055	Asparagus	82	Sausage	8
Arugula	1452	Celery	80	Figs	7
Spinach	1123	Watercress	73	Prunes	6
Chicory	938	Artichoke	63	Sweet potato	5
Wild radish	814	Eggplant	39	Raspberries	5
Bok choy	775	Strawberry	34	Raisins	4
Beet	632	Potato	26	Banana	4
Chinese cabbage	499	Garlic	19	Cherries	3
Beet (root) juice	482	Tomato	14	Onion	3
Lettuce	388	Vegetable juice	11	Red wine	3
Cabbage	312	Vegetable soup	10	Bean sprouts	2
Mustard greens	226	Cereal	10	Hot dog	1
Cauliflower, raw	167	Melon	10	Bacon	1
Parsley	150			Chickpeas	1
Kohlrabi	136			French fries	0
Carrot	127			Ham	0
Broccoli	122			Ketchup	0

The New, Nitrate-Based NO Supplement

Google the words "nitric oxide" and a lot of the results that instantly flash to the top of your computer screen are nitric oxide *supplements*—mostly being sold to body builders, and mostly with pumped up brand names featuring phrases such as "Professional Strength," "Overdrive," "Maximum Impact," "Stimulator," and "Force Factor."

Why are bodybuilders so excited about NO supplements?

According to an article at www.bodybuilding.com, "The fact that nitric oxide increases blood flow should make it of interest to bodybuilders, as increased blood flow will serve to deliver more nutrients to muscles, thus helping muscles become larger when subject to stress."

Well, we highly endorse any strategy that successfully helps bodybuilders, athletes, and fitness buffs boost their NO, through diet or supplements. (And, as you'll read in Chapter 4, on NO and exercise, new research shows that NO has the incredible ability to reduce your need for oxygen during exercise, and to a *greater* degree than you can achieve by training.)

However, we don't support the strategy employed by those NO-boosting supplements designed to help bodybuilders. Because those supplements boost NO (or at least try to boost NO) with L-arginine. That's okay if you're under 40 years old . . . and aren't overweight . . . and don't have high blood pressure . . . or diabetes . . . or high cholesterol . . . or smoke cigarettes. But if you're in any of those categories—and a lot of people, young, middle-aged, and old, are in those categories—your endothelium isn't going to effectively convert L-arginine to NO.

Let's look a little more closely at why NO-boosting supplements that rely on L-arginine aren't ideal.

The downside of L-arginine

L-arginine is an amino acid, one of the building blocks of protein. And it's a so-called *semi-essential amino acid:* your body doesn't manufacture all you need, so you have to get most of it from food. (It's mostly found in protein foods, such as red meat, fish, chicken, beans, and nuts.)

There's no question that L-arginine plays a key role in the formation of NO: enzymes called nitric oxide synthase (NOS) spark the oxidation of L-arginine to produce NO.

But that's a summary of what actually occurs. Biochemically, the L-arginine-to-NO pathway is very complex, with more than half a dozen compounds involved. And that's one of the main drawbacks of using an L-arginine supplement to boost NO levels in the body: the pathway requires L-arginine *and* other molecules; and if those molecules aren't on hand, L-arginine may make the situation worse. And that's just what some scientific studies show.

No help for peripheral arterial disease (PAD). Eight million Americans have the severe circulatory problem of PAD: clogged arteries in the legs that cause pain on walking (called *intermittent claudication*)—and a seven times higher risk of having a heart attack or stroke.

In a six-month study by doctors in the Division of Cardiovascular Medicine at Stanford University School of Medicine, 133 people with PAD took three grams of L-arginine a day or a placebo. The hoped-for benefit from the L-arginine supplement: the ability to walk farther without pain.

Well, those taking L-arginine supplements did have an increase in their blood levels of L-arginine. But that increase did *not* increase any of the standard measurements of NO production. There was no increase in "flow-mediated dilation," the NO-given ability of the arteries to widen. And there was no increase in blood levels of nitrate or nitrite, which turn into NO. In fact, in some study participants, those measurements *decreased.*

And after six months, the average improvement in walking distance of those taking L-arginine was *less* than in those taking the placebo: 11.5 percent for those taking L-arginine, compared to 28.3 percent for those taking the placebo. (The improvement in both groups was probably due to the placebo effect—because people think they're being given a medicine, they improve, even when they're taking a fake pill.)

"In patients with PAD, long-term administration of L-arginine does not increase nitric oxide synthesis or improve vascular reactivity [the ability of blood vessels to widen]," wrote the researchers in *Circulation*, the journal of the American Heart Association.

"Furthermore," they continued, "the data indicate that long-term administration of L-arginine may even impair functional capacity [the ability to walk without pain], perhaps through an adverse effect on vascular reactivity [the ability of blood vessels to widen]."

Why didn't L-arginine work? Why did it make the situation worse?

It might be due "to an arginine-induced derangement of the NOS pathway, with a paradoxical reduction in NO production," speculated the researchers.

And while they point out that many studies show a benefit from *short-term* use of L-arginine (one or two months), this benefit "is lost with long-term administration."

No protection after a heart attack. In another six-month study on L-arginine and cardiovascular disease, doctors in the Division of Cardiology at Johns Hopkins Medical Institutions and the Maryland Medical Research Institute studied 153 people after they had suffered a heart attack (myocardial infarction), giving half of them L-arginine (three grams, three times a day) and the other half a placebo.

To find out how L-arginine was working, they measured the strength and amount of the blood flow out of the heart (ejection fraction). They also measured the stiffness or flexibility of the arteries. And they kept track of how many people had another "cardiovascular event," such as angina or a heart attack. The results?

- L-arginine didn't improve ejection fraction compared to placebo.
- L-arginine didn't improve arterial stiffness compared to placebo.
- And six people in the L-arginine group *died*, compared to no one in the placebo group—at which point the doctors stopped the study, worried about the safety of L-arginine in people who had suffered a heart attack.

"L-arginine, when added to standard postinfarction therapies, does not improve vascular stiffness measurements or ejection fraction and may be associated with higher postinfarction mortality," concluded the researchers in the *Journal of the American Medical Association*. "L-arginine should not be recommended following acute myocardial infarction."

Also, the researchers noted that L-arginine will probably work to improve cardiovascular health only in people with "preexisting L-arginine deficiency" (such as people with chronic kidney disease, who can't metabolize protein or people who have elevated ADMA).

And they also noted that L-arginine is unlikely to work in people 60 and older, who have metabolic changes that inhibit their use of the amino acid. (The six people who died were all 60 years old or older.)

Why was L-arginine possibly harmful in older people who suffered a heart attack? "There are several potential mechanisms," wrote the researchers.

- The absence of NOS cofactors that guarantee the production of NOS—and without which L-arginine generates cell-damaging "reactive oxygen species" (free radicals).

- An L-arginine-caused increase in homocysteine, an amino acid linked to heart disease and stroke.
- And in people who have heart disease, L-arginine might actually spark the creation of too much NOS, thereby over-producing NO—and as you'll read in Chapter 6, too much NO can be as bad for you as too little.

"These potential consequences of L-arginine supplementation may explain, in part, the worse clinical outcomes in the older patients in this study randomized to L-arginine," wrote the researchers.

That study was published in January 2006. In 2009, Chinese researchers conducted a meta-analysis on studies using L-arginine after a heart attack, involving 927 people—and found the supplement didn't protect people from dying, compared to a placebo. "Oral L-arginine supplementation has no effect on the clinical outcomes of patients with acute myocardial infarction," concluded the researchers in the medical journal *Clinical Cardiology*.

Other no-result L-arginine studies. In a study in the *American Heart Journal* by researchers from the Hypertension and Vascular Disease Center at Wake Forest University School of Medicine, daily intake of food enriched with L-arginine (three grams) didn't improve endothelial function in people with high cholesterol.

Swedish researchers found that L-arginine supplements didn't improve arterial health after open heart surgery.

And in a two-month study by researchers at the National Heart, Lung, and Blood Institute of the National Institutes of Health, 30 people with heart disease took either L-arginine (nine grams daily) or a placebo—and L-arginine didn't improve "NO bioavailability." The results were in *Circulation*.

It's important to point out that many other scientific studies *do* show an improvement in cardiovascular health with L-arginine. L-arginine is a *possible* strategy for boosting NO. We just don't think it's the safest, most effective supplement strategy to increase NO in the patient population that can benefit the most from NO.

How to test your nitric oxide level

Your NO level won't shoot up and stay high—you constantly have to regenerate NO with moderate physical activity, food, supplements, and the other methods described in *The Nitric Oxide (NO) Solution*. Nitric Oxide Diagnostics Test Strips are a saliva-based test that allow you to see whether or not your NO-boosting strategy is actually boosting your NO levels.

First, test your baseline level of NO—the strip is color-coded, with faint pink showing a depleted level of NO and darker pink showing a normal level. This test can provide a quick answer to whether or not your NO restoration strategy is working. After taking a supplement or doing any NO-boosting activity, such as eating a spinach salad or going for a brisk walk, test your saliva 10 to15 minutes later, and again after 90-120 minutes. We now understand that people with endothelial dysfunction may not get the full benefit of exercise if they cannot make sufficient NO. Therefore exercise may or may not cause an increase in NO. Most recently we are beginning to understand the critical importance of oral bacteria in utilizing dietary nutrients to make NO. If you do not have the correct bacterial communities in the mouth and GI tract, you may not get the full benefit from your diet. The test strip will allow you to determine such limitations within your own body and then allow you to try different regimens that may work for you individually.

It's a wonderful way to make sure that your efforts to boost NO are actually working—and to give you confidence-building feedback when they are.

The Triglyceride Study

More proof of the power of nitric oxide: a scientific study conducted by Dr. Bryan, at the Center for Cell Signaling in the Institute of Molecular Medi¬cine at the University of Texas Health Science Center at Houston.

In his introduction to the study, Dr. Bryan makes his case for why a *different* strategy than L-arginine is called for.

"Remarkably," he writes, "strategies to restore NO homeostasis by supplementing L-arginine and antioxidants have consistently failed in clinical trials. This is due to the fact that the L-arginine-NO pathway is dysfunctional in patients with endothelial dysfunction." In other words, if you already have high blood pressure, advanced arterial plaque, or any form of cardiovascular disease, it's unlikely L-arginine is going to help you.

"In fact," he continues, "we now know that feeding the nitric oxide pathway through L-arginine supplementation may not always be effective and may be detrimental in at-risk patients."

He also notes that nitroglycerin (which works by boosting NO) is not an effective long-term strategy, because heart patients become tolerant to it and it stops working—and it even starts to hurt blood vessels.

In concluding his introduction, Dr. Bryan writes: "Despite NO's known and accepted importance in human physiology, there have been no hallmark therapeutic breakthroughs or effective strategies developed to enhance or restore NO homeostasis [normal levels of NO] in humans at risk for cardiovascular disease. Developing such strategies or technologies to restore and replete NO bioavailability is of paramount importance and could potentially save millions of lives worldwide and lessen the burden on the health care system."

"A daily regimen of reducing triglycerides and CRP and restoring NO homeostasis in patients with known cardiovascular disease risk factors is novel, with profound health implications," concludes Dr. Bryan.

NO-Boosting Recipes

These recipes were developed for us by Jennifer Adler, CN, a certified nutritionist and natural food chef in Seattle. She used high-NO foods on the NO Index—so you can eat these delicious meals knowing that you're giving your NO levels a *very* big boost.

The recipes are followed by a three-day meal plan that gives you examples of how to use the recipes for breakfasts, lunches, and dinners.

Enjoy!

Luscious Arugula and Dill Frittatas

Frittatas are a wonderful breakfast to make on the weekend. After they have cooled, you can place them in baggies and keep them in the fridge, to have throughout the rest of the week. This frittata starts your day off with a quick, grab-and-go, nutrient-dense breakfast that is packed with protein and NO-boosting green vegetables. They taste best reheated in a toaster oven.

Makes: 9 mini frittata "muffins" • Preparation time: 30–45 minutes

3 tablespoons butter or olive oil, divided

2 cloves garlic, minced

¼ cup diced red pepper

2 cups (2.5 ounces) chopped arugula

6 eggs

¼ cup heavy whipping cream

¼ teaspoon sea salt

¼ cup chopped fresh dill (or 2 tablespoons dried dill)

¾ cup grated Parmesan cheese

1. Preheat oven to 350°F.
2. Heat 2 tablespoons of butter in a medium-sized skillet over medium heat. Add garlic and cook for one to two minutes. Add red pepper and cook until the pepper is soft, about two to three minutes. Add the arugula and cook for one to two minutes, until wilted. Turn off the heat.
3. Prepare 9 muffin tin cups by oiling with remaining 1 tablespoon of butter or oil. In a large bowl, whisk eggs with the cream and salt. Fold the chopped dill, Parmesan, and arugula mixture into the eggs. Once it is incorporated, pour approximately ¼ cup into each of the 9 muffin cups. Place in the center of the oven and bake until the egg is firm in the middle, about 20–25 minutes.

Vibrant Tarragon and Beet Soup

This soup is a beautiful magenta color and is fabulous to have in the fall, winter, or for a special Valentine's treat. A wonderful way to add NO-boosting beets to your diet without the mess of peeling them, this soup freezes well so you can make a double batch for busy days ahead. Caramelizing the onion really adds depth to the soup. If you are not a tarragon fan, you can substitute basil or thyme. An alternative to the heavy cream is to use milk. Ume plum vinegar can be found in the vinegar or Asian section of a specialty grocery store. It has a salty, acidic flavor and is perfect for bringing soups or vegetables to life. When I was a personal chef, I would bring my knife and ume plum vinegar—because I knew I could fix any dish! If you cannot find ume plum vinegar, use apple cider vinegar instead.

Makes: 4 servings • Preparation time: 45 minutes

1½ tablespoons butter or olive oil

1 cup chopped onion

3 cups chopped beets

1 cup chopped apple

1 tablespoon sugar

¼ cup white wine

4 cups water or vegetable or chicken stock

1 teaspoon sea salt

¼ cup fresh tarragon (or 1½ tablespoons dried)

½ cup heavy cream

1½ tablespoons ume plum vinegar

4 tablespoons sour cream, for garnish (optional)

1. In a large stock pot, melt butter over medium heat. Add onion and sauté, stirring occasionally, until golden brown in color. Stir in beets and sauté for five minutes. Add apple and sugar and sauté one to two minutes, until the apple is soft.

2. Deglaze the pot by slowly pouring in the wine and scraping the stuck bits off the bottom of the pot with a wooden spoon. Add the stock and salt. Cover the pot and bring to a boil.

3. Reduce heat and let simmer until you can easily puncture the beets with a knife, about 25 minutes. Add tarragon, cream, and ume plum vinegar.

4. Use an immersion blender to puree the soup.

5. Serve in a bowl with a dollop of sour cream in the middle.

Crunchy Endive and Blue Cheese Salad

Curly endive, also called curly chicory, is a delicate vegetable with a powerful flavor. Radicchio is in the same family and provides a deliciously bitter quality often lacking in Western diets. If you are not a blue cheese fan, substitute feta. This is a bold salad that can be served as a side dish or as a topping for meat. It's hearty enough to last for a week in the refrigerator, although it will get softer and the color will fade as the days go by.

Makes: 4 main-dish servings or 8 side-dish servings • Preparation time: 15 minutes

2 garlic cloves, minced

4 cups (1 pound or 3 heads) chopped curly endive

1 cup (¼ pound or 1 small head) chopped radicchio

1 apple, chopped

1 cup toasted walnuts

1½ cup (4 ounces) crumbled blue cheese

3 tablespoons raw apple cider vinegar

¼ cup olive oil

1 teaspoon sea salt

1. In a medium-sized bowl, combine all ingredients.

Butter Lettuce Cups with Curried Chicken Salad

This is a tasty twist on the usual chicken salad. It utilizes lettuce instead of bread for a delicious, fresh lunch or snack. You can also use leftover chicken breast in place of the thighs.

Makes: 12 butter lettuce cups • Preparation time: 20 minutes

1½ pounds boneless, skinless chicken thighs

3 teaspoons curry powder

½ cup mayonnaise

4 tablespoons lemon juice (about 2 lemons)

3 tablespoons olive oil

2 teaspoons sea salt

1 cup toasted, chopped almonds

2 celery stalks, diced

⅓ cup chopped parsley

1 head butter leaf lettuce

1. Place chicken in a medium-sized saucepan. Cover with water and boil until the chicken is cooked through (165°F).
2. Remove from water and set aside to cool.
3. Once cooled, chop into small pieces.
4. In a medium-sized bowl, mix curry powder, mayonnaise, lemon juice, olive oil, and salt. Stir in chicken, almonds, celery, and parsley.
5. Serve ¼ cup chicken salad in each lettuce leaf. Fold the leaf over the chicken salad so it is easy to pick up and eat.

Crunchy Red Cabbage Slaw

This is a wonderful salad to make on the weekend, because it holds up well through the week. After you make it, portion it into individual containers for an easy-to-grab-in-the-morning vegetable to take with lunch. You can substitute green cabbage in place of red. This salad is also a potluck crowd-pleaser.

Makes: 4 servings • Preparation time: 20 minutes

3 cups chopped cabbage

½ teaspoon sea salt

½ cup halved cherry tomatoes

2 tablespoons lemon juice (about ½ lemon)

1 tablespoon olive oil

¼ cup chopped fresh basil

2 scallions, chopped

½ cup toasted sunflower seeds

1. Place cabbage in a large bowl. Sprinkle salt and massage into the cabbage for one minute.
2. Add the remaining ingredients and toss.

Creamy Wild Radish and Cucumber Salad

Wild radish is a different species from the cultivated radishes in our supermarkets, but it grows abundantly in the US. You can use the leaves like you would bok choy leaves. This salad holds up well for days. It is nice to have on hand to compliment fish or chicken, or to add to cottage cheese or a green salad. If the skin of the cucumber is too tough for you, it can be peeled.

Makes: 8 side-dish servings • Preparation time: 15 minutes

8 wild radish leaves, finely chopped

11 radishes, coarsely chopped

1 cucumber, seeded and chopped

2 teaspoons olive oil

2 tablespoons plus 1 teaspoon lemon juice

1¼ teaspoon sea salt

½ cup chopped fresh dill (or ¼ cup dried)

½ cup chopped parsley

¼ cup plain yogurt

1. Mix the above ingredients together in a bowl.

Chinese Cabbage and Chicken with Almond Sauce, Served over Coconut Quinoa

If you or your family likes Asian cuisine, this is likely to be a crowd pleaser. If you don't have any almond butter on hand, you can substitute peanut butter. Quinoa is a South American whole grain that is available in most grocery stores. It is a complete protein and cooks in about 15 minutes, making it ideal for busy schedules. If you have difficulty finding quinoa in your grocery store, you can use brown rice instead.

Makes: 4–6 servings • Preparation time: 40 minutes

1 cup vegetable or chicken stock

1 cup coconut milk

1 teaspoon sea salt

1⅓ cups quinoa

1½ pounds chicken breast

½ cup almond butter

½ cup orange juice

1 tablespoon grated ginger

3 garlic cloves, chopped

1 tablespoon maple syrup

6 tablespoons fish sauce

½ jalapeno, de-seeded and chopped (you can leave the seeds if you would like more spice)

1½ teaspoons sea salt

3 tablespoons toasted sesame oil

1 medium onion, chopped

4 cups chopped red cabbage

6 cups chopped Chinese cabbage

1 cup toasted, chopped almonds

3 tablespoons lime juice

1 cup chopped cilantro for garnish

1. Combine the stock, coconut milk, and salt in a one-quart saucepan over high heat and bring to a rapid boil.
2. Add the quinoa, cover, and lower the heat to a simmer.
3. Cook for 12 minutes, or until the water has been absorbed. The grain should be translucent and its thin germ/curlicue should be white.
4. Remove from the heat and let rest, covered for five minutes.
5. Fluff with a fork.
6. Place the chicken breasts into a large stock pot. Cover with water.
7. Boil until chicken is cooked through (165°F). Remove chicken from water. Set aside to cool.
8. Once it has cooled, shred chicken with a fork. Set aside.
9. Place the almond butter, orange juice, ginger, garlic, maple syrup, fish sauce, jalapeno, and salt in a blender and blend until smooth.
10. Place in a small saucepan and heat over medium-low heat.
11. Heat a large skillet or wok over medium-high and add sesame oil and onions.
12. Sauté until the onions are translucent.
13. Add cabbage and sauté until the cabbage has softened but is still crunchy, about five minutes.
14. Stir in chicken and sauté for three more minutes. Take off heat.
15. Stir in almonds and lime juice.
16. To serve, place quinoa on a plate. Serve cabbage and chicken mixture over the quinoa. Drizzle with the almond butter sauce and garnish with cilantro.

Sesame Halibut, Bok Choy, and Mango Stir-Fry, Served over Rice Noodles

The sweetness of the mango provides a fresh surprise in this dish. Whole wheat pastry flour is a good substitute for all-purpose flour and you can use it in almost any recipe. It has all of the vitamins, minerals, and fiber of whole wheat flour, but fries up light and fluffy, so it won't be detected by your family. If you don't have this available in your grocery store, however, you can use all-purpose flour.

Makes: 4–6 servings • Preparation time: 40 minutes

½ cup whole wheat pastry flour

Salt and pepper to taste

1 pound halibut steak, the skin and bones discarded, cut into ¾ inch pieces

¼ cup toasted sesame oil

2 cups chopped red onion

1½ tablespoons toasted sesame oil (if needed)

6 cups chopped bok choy

5 ounces frozen chopped mango

1 teaspoon sugar

2 teaspoons grated ginger

½ jalapeno, de-seeded and chopped (you can leave the seeds if you would like more spice)

3½ teaspoons rice vinegar

3½ teaspoons tamari or soy sauce

¼ teaspoon black pepper

2 tablespoons toasted sesame seeds

8 ounces of rice noodles, cooked according to package directions

1. In a small bowl, mix flour with salt and pepper. Dredge fish in flour mixture and tap off excess flour. Set aside.
2. In a large skillet heat oil over moderately high heat until it is hot, but not smoking. Fry the halibut in two batches. Cook on each side for one to two minutes, or until each is cooked through. Transfer with a slotted spoon to paper towels to drain.
3. Add red onion to remaining sesame oil in skillet (add more oil if there is no more in the skillet). Sauté onion until translucent over medium-high heat. Add bok choy, mango, sugar, ginger,

jalapeno, rice vinegar, tamari, and pepper and sauté until bok choy is soft but still crunchy, about two to three minutes. Remove from heat. Sprinkle with sesame seeds.

4. Serve by placing rice noodles on a plate with bok choy served over it and halibut on the top.

Mediterranean Spinach and Quinoa Salad

If a fine mesh strainer is not part of your kitchen equipment, you can cook the quinoa in a pot with 1 cup quinoa and 2 cups liquid for 13 minutes, or until the liquid is absorbed. If you don't have quinoa available in your grocery store, you can use brown rice instead. This salad is great to have on hand for easy-to-make lunches because it lasts for 5–10 days in the fridge.

Makes: 4–6 servings • Preparation time: 30 minutes

8 cups water

1 cup quinoa

5 cups chopped spinach

½ teaspoon salt

½ cup chopped sun-dried tomatoes

6 tablespoons olive oil

4 tablespoons lemon juice

½ cup chopped red bell pepper

½ cup chopped green or kalamata olives

1½ teaspoons salt

½ cup diced red onion

1 cup crumbled feta

1 cup cooked garbanzo beans

½ cup toasted pine nuts

1. Bring water to a boil in a large stock pot over high heat. As water comes to a boil, toast quinoa in a large skillet over medium heat until browned. Once water boils, slowly add

the toasted quinoa. Reduce heat and simmer for 13 minutes. Strain through a fine mesh strainer and set aside.

2. In a large bowl mix spinach with salt. Stir until spinach wilts. Stir in remaining ingredients. *Gently* fold in quinoa. Serve chilled.

Velvet Mustard Greens

The texture and flavor of mustard greens is made palatable to even the pickiest eaters by boiling it first, which makes it mild, soft, and velvety. This is a nice side dish to bring for a holiday dinner. Try reheating leftovers for breakfast with a fried egg on top.

Makes: 4 servings • Preparation time: 30 minutes

1 pound mustard greens, tough stems and center ribs discarded and leaves cut into 1-inch-wide strips (4 cups)

3 tablespoons butter

1 small red onion, halved lengthwise and thinly sliced crosswise

3 garlic cloves, minced

1 tablespoon red-wine vinegar, or to taste

¼ teaspoon salt

1. Cook mustard greens in a six-quart pot of boiling water, uncovered, stirring occasionally, until just tender, about 10 minutes. Drain in a colander.

2. Heat butter in a 12-inch heavy skillet over moderately high heat until hot, but not smoking. Add onion and sauté, stirring occasionally, until softened, about six to eight minutes. Add garlic and sauté, stirring, until garlic is fragrant, about one minute. Reduce heat to medium, then add mustard greens and cook, stirring occasionally, until heated through. Remove from heat and stir in vinegar and salt.

Raw Beet Salad

This is a power-packed nitrate-rich salad that will help your body generate a large amount of NO. This tasty mixture will also keep for several days in the fridge—make it on a weekend to have on hand for a busy week.

Makes: 4–6 servings • Preparation time: 10 minutes

1 beet, shredded (make sure the beets are firm and still sweet)

1 carrot, shredded

1 green apple (or apple of your choice), shredded

½ cup red cabbage, shredded

1 tablespoon lemon juice

1 teaspoon ume plum vinegar (or apple cider vinegar)

1 tablespoon of olive oil

Freshly ground black pepper to taste

1. Mix all ingredients together and serve. You can also add scallions, red onion, or your favorite fresh herbs.

Fresh Green Cashew-Walnut Pate

This vegan pate is rich in NO-boosting nitrate and nitrite, and also in heart-healthy omega-3 oils. Feel free to substitute other nuts for the cashews and walnuts (such as brazil nuts, almonds, sunflower seeds, or pumpkin seeds). You can also use any fresh leafy green in place of the kale—pick your favorite.

Makes: 4–6 servings • Preparation time: 10–15 minutes

6 ounces raw unsalted cashews

2 ounces raw walnuts

1 handful parsley

2 leaves fresh kale

1 lime or lemon, juiced

¼ teaspoon natural salt (Celtic sea salt, Himalayan salt)

NO-Boosting

Three-Day Meal Plan

This meal plan features some of the NO-boosting recipes in *The Nitric Oxide (NO) Solution*, along with other foods high on the NO Index.

DAY ONE

Breakfast: Luscious Arugula and Dill Frittatas

Snack: Celery and Almond Butter (or Peanut Butter)

Lunch: Butter Lettuce Cups with Curried Chicken Salad

Snack: Blanched Cauliflower, Broccoli, and Raw Carrots with Hummus

Dinner: Vibrant Tarragon and Beet Soup with Toasted Sprouted Grain Bread with Butter

DAY TWO

Breakfast: Miso Soup with Bok Choy and Eggs or Cubed Tofu (*Note:* You can crack the eggs into the broth when it is heating and stir it to have an egg drop soup effect. Then stir in chopped bok choy and miso. To make it even heartier, you can add leftover brown rice.)

Snack: Beet Chips (can be purchased at specialty grocery stores)

Lunch: Mediterranean Spinach and Quinoa Salad

Snack: Butter Lettuce Cups with Crunchy Endive and Blue Cheese Salad

Dinner: Sesame Halibut, Bok Choy, and Mango Stir-Fry, Served over Rice Noodles

DAY THREE

Breakfast: Velvet Mustard Greens with a Fried Egg served on top and Toasted Sprouted Grain Bread

Snack: Smoothie (*Note:* Blend a banana, frozen berries, fresh spinach, yogurt, and milk or juice until smooth. You will not notice the spinach.)

Lunch: Crunchy Red Cabbage Slaw with Leftover Chicken or Canned White Beans

Snack: Butter Lettuce Cups with Creamy Wild Radish and Cucumber Salad

Dinner: Chinese Cabbage and Chicken with Almond Sauce, Served over Coconut Quinoa

Freshly ground black pepper to taste

Granulated garlic to taste

Seasoning of your choice (such as dill, turmeric, Thai kitchen curry paste, teaspoon of white miso) to taste

1. Process all ingredients in a Cuisinart, Vita Mix, or any food processor, to a smooth pate consistency.
2. Serve on celery sticks, lettuce leaves, inside a bell pepper, etc.

FOUR

NO-Sweat: Easy Exercises to Enhance NO

Can You Spare 11 Minutes to Save Your Life?

Let's start this chapter with a simple and important fact.

If you exercise—if you take a brisk walk or jog, if you bike or swim, if you jump rope or do jumping jacks, if you do *anything* for 10 minutes or longer that raises your heart rate a bit and keeps it raised—you're going to produce more health-giving NO.

A Refresher Course in the Endothelium

To understand how exercise generates NO, let's take a quick refresher course, revisiting some of the information you read in Chapter 1, when you first learned about how NO works.

The endothelium is the lining of the blood vessels, and it makes NO.

NO is a messenger molecule: it tells the blood vessels to dilate—to widen—like an expandable tunnel that allows more traffic to pass through.

With enough NO, the blood vessels relax and widen.

With enough NO, blood flows from and to the healthy heart.

With enough NO, there's less risk of the toxic buildup of artery-clogging plaque.

With enough NO, there's normal blood pressure levels, because arteries aren't tense and tight.

With enough NO, there's less risk of heart attack and stroke.

But when you don't have enough NO, the endothelium begins to work poorly, which is the first step in *atherosclerosis*, the hardening and clogging of the arteries that can lead to a heart attack and stroke.

Without enough NO, you have high blood pressure . . . the stressed endothelium is weakened and cracked . . . cholesterol sticks in the cracks, causing wound-like inflammation . . . the immune system is alerted and rushes white blood cells to the area . . . they also stick to the NO-poor endothelium . . . the mixture of cholesterol and dead white blood cells begins the buildup of plaque . . . eventually, the plaque ruptures and spills its contents into the bloodstream . . . a blood clot is formed—and you have a heart attack or stroke!

NO is produced in the arteries by an enzyme called endothelial nitric oxide synthase, or eNOS.

Exercise boosts eNOS. And (a remarkable new finding) more NO also boosts your capacity to exercise!

In this chapter, we'll look at four major areas having to do with NO and exercise: (1) research showing that exercise boosts NO; (2) research showing that more NO helps you exercise; (3) research showing that exercise protects the heart; and (4) a discussion of the whys and wherefores of an exercise program—and exactly how much exercise you need to get the NO-boosting benefits. (It's not much: an average of 22 minutes a day does the trick, and that could be *two* 11-minute walks.)

The NO-Exercise Link

The link between NO and exercise is what scientists like to call *bidirectional*:

- Exercise improves your ability to produce NO.
- NO improves your ability to exercise.

Let's look at both sides of that equation.

Exercise improves your ability to produce NO

"Regular physical activity has a strong positive link with cardiovascular health," wrote a team of researchers from the University of Missouri–

Columbia, in a review of decades of scientific literature on exercise and the heart. But *how* does it have a positive effect?

Exercise speeds up blood flow, which keeps the endothelium toned, washes away inflammation, stops blood from becoming sludge-like, and prevents the buildup of artery-clogging plaque.

And, say the researchers, that increased blood flow *also* stimulates the endothelium's production of NO—which keeps blood pressure low, and helps stop cholesterol from attaching itself to artery walls and starting the formation of plaque.

Here are some of the studies on the link between NO, exercise, and cardiovascular health.

Exercise generates NO—and improves blood flow. Noting that "aerobic exercise enhances endothelium-dependent vasodilation [widening of the arteries] in healthy people, people with high blood pressure, and people with congestive heart failure," a team of Japanese researchers conducted a study to find out *why.*

They tested 26 healthy young men, asking them to ride on a stationary bike for 30 minutes, five to seven times a week, at different intensity levels (mild, moderate, and high). After three months, the men in the moderate-intensity group had a greater degree of blood flow in their forearms (a standard scientific measurement for increased endothelial health and improved circulation). But when the researchers injected the men with a compound that stopped the formation of eNOS, the level of blood flow returned to what it was in the months before they exercised—clear proof that it was NO that made the flow-increasing difference.

"Moderate-intensity aerobic exercise augments endothelium-dependent vasodilation in humans through the increased production of nitric oxide," concluded the researchers in the medical journal *Circulation.*

Interestingly, the researchers found that low-intensity exercise wasn't intense enough to improve blood flow, and that high-intensity exercise worsened blood flow, probably because it generated excess, cell-damaging oxidative stress.

Moderation in all things—including everyday exercise!

In a similar study, in the *American Journal of Hypertension,* Japanese researchers noted that "long-term moderate-intensity exercise augments endothelium-dependent vasodilation through an increase in NO production." And like their colleagues, they found that moderate-intensity exercise worked best.

Exercise lowers high blood pressure—because it boosts NO. In another study from Japan, 20 people with high blood pressure were divided into two groups: 10 exercised regularly for three months, and 10 didn't. After three months, there was increased blood flow in the forearms of the exercisers—an increase that could be "abolished" by the compound that stops the production of eNOS.

"Long-term physical exercise improves endothelium-dependent vasorelaxation through an increase in release of nitric oxide in . . . hypertensive subjects," concluded the researchers in the journal *Circulation*.

High cholesterol levels can't stop exercise from boosting NO. Australian researchers studied nine sedentary people with high cholesterol, asking them to start using a stationary bike for 30 minutes, three times a week. After one month, the group had an average 6 percent higher blood level of nitrate and nitrite, the precursors of NO. (Their blood pressure also dropped.)

"Endothelium-derived NO is increased with 4 weeks of home training in hypercholesterolemic [high cholesterol] patients," concluded the researchers in the journal *Arteriosclerosis, Thrombosis, and Vascular Biology*. "This may contribute to the cardiovascular effects of exercise training, including reduced blood pressure."

Stop the NO—stop the exercise-improved flow. In a study by researchers at the National Institutes of Health, 18 healthy but sedentary people (average age 40) started exercising—and the blood flow in their forearms increased. But when the eNOS-blocking drug was given, that blood flow was reduced—and the higher the dose of the drug, the greater the reduction in blood flow.

"Inhibition of nitric oxide synthesis reduces exercise-induced vasodilation," concluded the researchers, in the journal *Circulation*.

NO decreases with age—but not if you exercise! As you age, your endothelium ages, too: your arteries become tighter and less flexible, and your risk for heart disease and stroke increases. A big reason for that change is (you guessed it) your NO production decreases as you age. Exercise can help prevent that from happening!

In a study on exercise, NO, and aging, Italian researchers studied four groups:

1. Young sedentary (average age 27)
2. Old sedentary (average age 63)
3. Young athletes (average age 27)
4. Old athletes (average age 66)

They measured the forearm blood flow in all four groups, and then gave them an eNOS-inhibiting drug. The blood flow of the old athletes remained much stronger than the blood flow of the old sedentary group.

"Regular physical activity can at least in part prevent age-induced endothelial dysfunction, probably because of the restoration of nitric oxide availability," concluded the researchers in the journal *Circulation*.

A similar study was conducted by researchers in the Human Cardiovascular Research Laboratory at the Center for Physical Activity, Disease Prevention, and Aging at the University of Colorado.

They conducted an experiment with 68 healthy men in the same four categories: young sedentary and young exerciser (22 to 35 years old) and older sedentary and older exerciser (50 to 76 years old).

Among the older sedentary men, the eNOS-blocking drug reduced forearm blood flow. But the same drug had no effect on the older exercisers—who had the same flow as the younger exercisers!

Then the researchers put the sedentary men on a three-month exercise program (mostly regular walking)—and their blood flow increased by 30 percent, to the levels of the younger and older exercisers. (It's *never* too late to start exercising!)

"Regular aerobic exercise can prevent the age-associated loss in endothelium dependent vasodilation and restore levels in previously sedentary middle aged and older healthy men," concluded the researchers in the journal *Circulation*.

NO improves your ability to exercise

Okay, that's a scientific lock: there's no doubt that exercise boosts NO. But recent research also shows that providing extra NO—through diet, supplements, or other means—also boosts your capacity to exercise. Let's take a look at this remarkable scientific finding.

Eat beets—and exercise longer, with less effort. Researchers from the University of Exeter in the UK studied eight men (ages 19 to 38). Every day for three days (Days 1, 2, and 3 of the study), the men drank either 17 ounces (500 ml) of nitrate-rich beet juice or a look-alike placebo drink. (Remember: nitrate turns into NO and beet is high on the NO Index.)

Then, on the last three days of the study (Days 4, 5, and 6), the men exercised at either a moderate or severe intensity level.

The beet-drinkers couldn't be beat.

Those who drank the beet juice had 49 percent higher levels of nitrite in their blood.

Their blood pressure was 6 percent lower than that of the placebo group—even though they didn't have high blood pressure to start with.

And during moderate exercise, the muscles of the beet-drinkers required 19 percent less oxygen to perform the same task—a sure sign of increased muscular efficiency.

The beet group could also exercise 16 percent longer without becoming exhausted. (The beet goes on!)

The researchers were amazed at the results, describing them as "remarkable"—which, in the staid pages of scientific journals, is a word one rarely sees. The quote:

"It should be stressed that the remarkable reduction in the O_2 [oxygen] cost of sub-maximal exercise following dietary supplementation with inorganic nitrate in the form of a natural food product [the beets] cannot be achieved by any other known means, including long-term endurance exercise training," concluded the researchers in the *Journal of Applied Physiology*.

In other words, boosting your NO by eating beets is *more* effective than endurance training in making your body more efficient during exercise! So if you want to train for any sports activity, eat lots of NO-producing beets—or any other food high on the NO Index.

Or if you want to train for life.

"In certain human populations (including the senescent [elderly] and those with cardiovascular, respiratory or metabolic diseases [such as diabetes]), the activities of daily living are physically difficult because they have an energy requirement that requires" a lot of lung power, wrote the researchers. "A reduction in needed oxygen . . . associated with such activities following dietary nitrate supplementation therefore has the potential to improve exercise tolerance and the quality of life in these groups."

In other words, if you have heart disease . . . or have had a stroke . . . or have chronic obstructive pulmonary disease . . . or asthma . . . or are aging . . . or have type 2 diabetes . . . or if you have *any* problem that impedes your ability to move around without some degree of muscular stress and strain and breathlessness—increasing your NO is a really, really good idea!

It's important to note that the "remarkable" result we presented was also produced in another study by a team of scientists from the prestigious Karolinska Institute of Sweden—the "replication" of findings that is the test of the truth of any scientific discovery.

"Dietary nitrate supplementation, in an amount achievable through a diet rich in vegetables, results in a lower oxygen demand" during exercise, concluded the researchers in the medical journal *Acta Physiologica*.

And in a study of 55 people, researchers from Germany found that exercise increased blood levels of NO-forming nitrite by 22 percent—that the more nitrite a person formed, the harder and longer they could exercise. The findings were in the *British Journal of Sports Medicine*.

Exercise and Cardiovascular Disease (CVD)

If exercise is NO-boosting and endothelium-healing, then it should help prevent or reverse the circulatory problems collectively known as *cardiovascular disease* (CVD).

Once again, scientific studies show that's exactly what happens when you exercise regularly. Here is some of the most recent research:

Exercise prevents CVD. "Habitual physical activity [such as walking, running, or swimming] prevents the development of coronary artery disease [CAD]," says a "scientific statement" from the American Heart Association titled "Exercise and Physical Activity in the Prevention and Treatment of Atherosclerotic Cardiovascular Disease."

What Allows Tibetans to Live and Work at High Altitudes? Four Times More NO!

An international team of researchers from the Cleveland Clinic, the Boston University School of Medicine, Ohio State University, and other institutions measured NO levels in two groups: 88 Tibetans living at 13,780 feet above sea level (4,200 meters) and 50 Americans living at sea level.

The Americans were NO-challenged.

The Tibetans had more than *double* the forearm blood flow of the Americans. They also had 10 times more bioactive NO products in their blood, including nitrate and nitrite ("remarkably high levels," observed the researchers). And they had a fourfold higher production of NO.

"This suggests that NO production is increased and that metabolic pathways controlling formation of NO products are regulated differently among Tibetans," concluded the researchers in the *Proceedings of the National Academy of Sciences*.

If you're planning on any situation that will require more oxygen—such as more exercise, or high-altitude traveling, or the (unplanned) oxygen-demanding stress of most severe illnesses—increase your NO!

They continue: 50 years of "studies of occupational and leisure-time physical activity have consistently documented a reduced incidence of CAD events [such as angina, heart attack, heart surgery, and heart failure] in the more physically active and fit."

Yes, it's *that* simple and straightforward: regular exercise keeps your arteries healthy.

And remember, CVD isn't only about heart attacks—it's about heart attacks *and* strokes. Exercise prevents both.

Prevent a stroke—with exercise. In an analysis of 40 studies on physical activity and stroke, a team of German researchers found that regular exercise reduced stroke risk by 32 percent. "Physical activity is found to have a protective effect" against stroke, concluded the researchers.

Research also shows exercise can lower CVD risk factors *after* a stroke. In a study by doctors at the University of Illinois, 55 stroke survivors were enrolled in various types of 14-week exercise programs. Exercise lowered blood pressure, lowered total cholesterol, and lowered triglycerides—resulting in "coronary risk reduction," concluded the researchers in the *Archives of Physical Medicine and Rehabilitation.*

That's right—exercise doesn't only *prevent* CVD. It also slows, stops, and even reverses it.

Increase exercise, lower blood pressure. Noting that studies show "blood pressure is lower in individuals who are more fit and active," a team of Belgian cardiologists reviewed 72 studies on aerobic exercise and hypertension, involving nearly four thousand people.

On average, exercise reduced blood pressure by 3 points systolic and 2.4 points diastolic.

For people *with* hypertension, exercise reduced pressure by 7 points systolic and 5 points diastolic.

And in 12 studies, resistance training (also called strength training or muscle training, and involving weights, bands, or other forms of resistance) reduced systolic pressure an average of 3.2 and diastolic an average of 3.5 points.

In another study on exercise and hypertension, researchers at Duke University Medical Center added exercise to the regimen of hypertensives eating the healthy, pressure-lowering DASH diet (Dietary Approaches to Stop Hypertension). And their blood pressure fell even more: an average 11/8 point decline with the DASH diet changed to an average 16/10 point decline with the DASH diet *and* exercise.

Fats get fit, too. When blood fats are tested, the best results are (in milligrams per deciliter, or mg/dL):

- low "bad" LDL cholesterol (less than 100)
- low total cholesterol (less than 200)
- high "good" HDL cholesterol (60 and above)
- low triglycerides (less than 150)

Well, fitness trims your fat, outside *and* in.

In a review of cholesterol-lowering factors in the journal *American Family Physician*, a doctor from the Cleveland Clinic notes that "regular aerobic exercise has beneficial effects on lipid [blood fat] levels, particularly if performed at least 120 minutes per week."

In a study of 77 women 60 to 79 years old, researchers in Portugal found that a combination of exercises—aerobic, muscle training, balance, and stretching—effectively lowered triglycerides by 5.1 percent and increased HDL by 9.3 percent.

Other studies show that exercise boosts HDL—in fact, that it's one of the *best* ways to boost it.

Researchers at the University of Wisconsin studied 26 nonexercising, postmenopausal women, dividing them into three groups: (1) 45 minutes of exercise, five days a week; (2) 30 minutes of exercise, five days a week; and (3) no exercise. The more the women exercised, the higher their boost in HDL. The study also found that the 45-minute exercisers had more weight loss and took more inches off their waists.

The latest thinking about LDL cholesterol and heart disease—it's very *small, dense* particles of LDL (compared to big, fluffy particles) that do the most damage. The tiny, toxic particles are called apolipoprotein B (ApoB). And in a 17-month study by Japanese researchers, people who started an exercise program also lowered ApoB—and the fitter they were, the lower their ApoB. They also had drops in blood pressure, triglycerides, weight, and waist size.

Cooling chronic inflammation. C-reactive protein (CRP) is a biomarker for chronic low-grade inflammation and a risk factor for heart disease. In a study by Australian researchers, 102 nonexercisers were divided into three groups: (1) 41 people started an aerobic exercise program; (2) 35 people started a muscle-training program; and (3) 26 people didn't do anything. After 10 weeks, CRP was reduced in the aerobic group by 16 percent and in the muscle-training group by 33 percent.

Recovering from heart disease—with exercise. Cardiac rehabilitation is standard therapy after a heart attack or medical procedure to open blocked arteries, and it's always "exercise-based"—that is, exercise is the main therapy.

Noting that cardiac rehabilitation programs reduce future heart attacks and death rates from heart disease, a team of Japanese researchers studied 111 older (65 and older) people with heart disease, some who participated in cardiac rehabilitation and some who didn't.

Those participating had 57 percent fewer "cardiovascular events" (angina, heart attacks, angiography procedures to open blocked arteries, congestive heart failure, and strokes) and a 14 percent lower death rate.

And in a study in the *American Journal of Health Promotion*, researchers looked at 24 cardiac rehabilitation programs in the US, involving nearly three thousand people. After three months, the participants had lower:

- LDL cholesterol
- total cholesterol
- triglycerides, a heart-harming blood fat
- diastolic blood pressure
- systolic blood pressure
- hemoglobin A1c, a measure of long-term blood sugar control (high blood sugar is a risk factor for CVD)
- weight
- depression (a risk factor for heart disease)
- hostility (another risk factor)

Not bad for the heart-healing effects of regular exercise!

Controlling congestive heart failure. Heart disease (particularly a heart attack) can damage and weaken the heart muscle so much that its pumping power is compromised—you're short of breath, tired, weak, and may have swollen feet and legs.

This is called congestive heart failure (CHF)—and exercise can make it a lot better.

UK researchers analyzed data from 19 studies on exercise and CHF, involving more than 3,600 people. It showed that exercise improved the ability to exercise, reduced hospital admissions for CHF, and improved quality of life (the ability to engage in and enjoy everyday activities).

And in one recent study in the journal *Circulation: Heart Failure*, German researchers found that three months of regular exercise strengthened the hearts of CHF patients, including improving blood flow, "suggestive of improvement of endothelial function."

Intermittent claudication—exercise eases the leg pain. Arteries don't only become narrow and clogged around your heart. You can also develop *peripheral arterial disease* (PAD)—clogged arteries in your legs. And the primary symptom in PAD is *intermittent claudication*—severe pain in your leg muscles when you walk. But walking isn't only the cause of intermittent claudication. It's also the cure.

A team of Irish researchers analyzed 23 studies on intermittent claudication and exercise, and found that an exercise program could reduce pain and improve walking distance.

And in a study by Dutch researchers of 304 people with intermittent claudication, exercise therapy improved walking distance before pain by nearly one-quarter mile.

Solving the metabolic syndrome. The metabolic syndrome is a constellation of conditions that can include high blood sugar, overweight with excess abdominal fat, high triglycerides, high blood pressure, high LDL, and low HDL—and it's a risk factor for heart disease and stroke. Exercise can help bring it under control.

Austrian researchers analyzed the results of 13 studies on the metabolic syndrome and muscle training, and found that muscle training helped reduce obesity, high blood sugar levels, and high blood pressure, and "should be recommended in the management" of the metabolic syndrome.

In another study, doctors at the Case Western Reserve University School of Medicine in Cleveland asked 24 people with the metabolic syndrome to go on an exercise program. Exercise improved blood sugar levels, lowered blood pressure, slimmed waists, lowered LDL, and lowered triglycerides.

"Exercise alone is an effective nonpharmacological treatment strategy for metabolic syndrome and cardiovascular risk factors," concluded the researchers in the *Journal of Gerontology: Biological Sciences.*

Exercise works no matter how old you are. Researchers at the University of British Columbia in Vancouver studied the effect of exercise on people usually considered too far gone for exercise to make any difference: people 70 years old with type 2 diabetes (which doubles the risk of heart disease and stroke), high blood pressure, and high cholesterol. But after three months of aerobic exercise—walking on a treadmill or exercising on a stationary bike a couple of times a week—the study participants had arteries that were far more flexible and youthful.

"A relatively short aerobic exercise intervention in older adults can reduce arterial stiffness," concluded the researchers in the journal *Diabetes Care.*

Or how young. Unfortunately, it's not just adults who are at risk for heart disease. Many of today's kids—overweight and sedentary—have the full range of cardiovascular risk factors, including high cholesterol, high blood pressure, and high triglycerides.

In a study of 51 overweight kids aged 6 to 12, participation in four months of exercise (three 60-minute sessions a week) significantly improved blood pressure, LDL levels, and triglycerides, along with waist size, muscle mass, and lung capacity.

And in a study in the *International Journal of Pediatric Obesity* (yes, there *is* such a journal, which gives you an idea of the scope of the problem), researchers at West Virginia University found that when 35 overweight 10-year-olds regularly exercised using the *Dance Dance Revolution* video game, they had significant improvements in blood flow, with 13 of the kids achieving "normal endothelial function" after three months.

How Much Should You Exercise?

There are *so* many benefits to regular exercise besides a healthier cardiovascular system. Studies show regular exercise can help prevent, treat, or lessen the symptoms of:

- AIDS
- Alzheimer's disease
- anxiety
- asthma
- arthritis
- cancer
- chronic fatigue syndrome
- chronic obstructive pulmonary disease (COPD)
- colds and flu
- depression
- diabetes

- falls
- fibromyalgia
- gallstones
- insomnia
- low back pain
- menopausal symptoms, such as hot flashes
- multiple sclerosis
- osteoporosis
- overweight
- stress

But *how much* exercise—how many minutes a week, and at what level of intensity—really prevents and treats disease?

It's not so easy to know.

There are so *many* recommendations out there for the *amount* of weekly exercise that you need; you may have become confused. And why wouldn't you be?

There are exercise recommendations from the Office of the Surgeon General . . . the National Institutes of Health . . . the US Department of Agriculture . . . the Department of Health and Human Services . . . the Institute of Medicine . . . the American College of Sports Medicine . . . and many other governmental and public organizations. And for the most part, they're all different!

To clear up the confusion, we talked with David Neiman, PhD, director of the Human Performance Lab at the North Carolina Research Campus, and author of *Exercise Testing and Prescription*, the leading textbook for physical education teachers, coaches, and others who want to learn how to help people improve their health with exercise.

Dr. Neiman told us that, finally, there are straightforward, practical, and accurate guidelines for the amount of physical activity you need for "health, fitness, and disease prevention."

The guidelines are the *2008 Physical Activity Guidelines for Americans* (PA Guidelines), from the Department of Health and Human Services and the US Department of Agriculture.

Here are those specific guidelines, courtesy of Dr. Neiman and the

Health and Fitness Journal of the American College of Sports Medicine (ACSM):

All adults should avoid inactivity. Some physical activity is better than none, and adults who participate in *any* amount of physical activity gain some health benefits.

The best level for "substantial" health benefits. Here's the number you've been waiting for: 150 minutes a week of moderate-intensity physical activity, such as a brisk walk. A 30-minute walk, five days a week, fulfills your goal!

Or divide 150 (minutes) by seven (days a week), and the result is 21 or 22 minutes per day. Take two 11-minute walks every day—about six minutes out and six minutes back—and you've met (and even slightly exceeded) the goal! That is *not* much exercise for health and actual healing!

You can tell you're doing moderate-intensity physical activity when you raise your heart rate above resting rate, and when you break a sweat. You're able to talk—but your lungs are challenged enough that you're not able to sing the words to a song. Brisk walking is moderate intensity (and the most popular exercise among those who exercise regularly).

Other examples of moderate-intensity activity from the government's Centers for Disease Control and Prevention (CDC) include:

- doing water aerobics
- riding a bike on level ground or with few hills
- playing doubles tennis
- pushing a lawn mower

If you want to workout less than 150 minutes a week, you have to workout harder: 75 minutes a week of vigorous-intensity physical activity, such as jogging or playing singles tennis. At this level of activity, you're breathing hard and fast, and your heart is pumping really hard. You can't say more than a few words without pausing for breath.

Other examples of vigorous-intensity activity include:

- jogging or running
- swimming laps

- riding a bike fast or on hills
- playing singles tennis
- playing basketball

If you're mixing and matching moderate- and vigorous-intensity activity, think of the two-for-one rule—every minute of vigorous activity equals two minutes of moderate intensity.

So if you play a 30-minute pickup basketball game with your buddies, you still need 45 more minutes of vigorous-intensity activity to meet your goal—or 90 more minutes of moderate activity.

10 minutes is the minimum. Less than 10 minutes won't get your heart pumping at a level where the health benefits kick in. But 10 minutes at a time *is* perfectly okay—and that's not a whole lot of time!

Seniors are covered. These same guidelines apply to adults 65 and over, Dr. Neiman told us. But, he said, you should adapt them as your "abilities and conditions allow." In other words, if you've got severe knee osteoarthritis, it might be hard to meet the guidelines.

We'd like to point out, however, that working out in a warm pool is *perfect* for people with chronic and painful diseases that limit their exercise. In one study from Danish researchers, published in the journal *Physical Therapy*, people with knee or hip osteoarthritis who exercised in the water for six weeks had less joint pain, stiffness, and got around more easily during the day. Studies also show that water exercise can help: with fibromyalgia (chronic, body-wide muscle pain); with recovering after knee replacement surgery; in reducing the swelling of lymphedema after breast surgery for cancer; and stop the bone loss of pre-osteoporosis (osteopenia) or osteoporosis.

Balance is important, too. Every year, more than 30 percent of people age 65 and over *fall*—with 1 in 10 seriously injured, and nearly 30 thousand killed. That's why the PA Guidelines urge older adults to do exercises that "maintain or improve balance if they are at risk of falling," said Dr. Neiman. The best exercises for improving balance: walking, dancing, muscle training, and tai chi.

Guidelines for the disabled. "When adults with disabilities are not able to meet these activity guidelines, they should engage in regular physical activity according to their abilities, and avoid inactivity," Dr. Neiman told us.

"Die Young at a Very Old Age"

Words of Wisdom on Exercise and Longevity, from Vikram Khanna, CES

Whenever we want to find out the straight (and scientific) scoop on exercise and health, we like to talk to Vikram ("Vik") Khanna, a Clinical Exercise Specialist certified by the American College of Sports Medicine (ACSM), and the self-described "Chief Exercise Officer" of Galileo Health Partners near Baltimore, Maryland. (You can read Vik's superb blog, and find your way from there to his website, at http://galileohealth.net/blog.) Recently, we asked Vik to share his perspective on extending your life through exercise. He pointed us to a recent post on the subject, which we've reprinted most of here. Vik begins:

Most people estimate their likely lifespan using two parallel measures: how long they think they might live and how well they live (also called quality of life). While most people want to live a long life, many understand that living a high quality of life may actually matter more. Living longer, but suffering because of disease or disability, is not enticing, while aiming to "die young at a very old age" encompasses a more robust vision of living better and, hopefully, longer.

The essence of both *better* life and *longer* life is *lifestyle*; the better your choices, the more likely you are to achieve your goals of living better and longer. A healthy lifestyle is the ultimate, dual-purpose life preserver because it will empower you to live better today (happier, stronger, less stressed) and give you the best chance at abundant tomorrows.

The critical lifestyle factors, based on our understanding today, are:

- body composition (expressed as body weight, waistline, or body mass index [BMI])
- physical activity
- fruit/vegetable/alcohol consumption
- smoking

[An aside from Vik's excellent commentary: we'd like to note that increasing your physical activity, eating more vegetables and fruits, and not smoking have something in common: they all increase NO!]

These, in turn, affect important clinical measures, such as blood pressure, glucose/insulin metabolism, blood lipids, and inflammation. When these measures worsen, disease results.

Of the lifestyle factors, smoking is the easiest to dissect. In studies, smoking increases the death rate by two to three times. In lifestyle analyses, stopping smoking is generally considered *the* most important and powerful lifestyle step you can take.

After smoking, a high level of physical fitness offers *unparalleled* protective effects.

A highly fit person (along with not smoking and eating enough fruit/vegetables) may be *12 to 14 years younger* than a physically unfit person with bad habits. In other words, the fit person's body has healthy, youthful characteristics (such as lower blood pressure and healthier blood vessels) that persist even during the aging process. This is important because many measures of health risk, such as rising blood pressure and cardiac dysfunction, get worse with age.

Research also shows that being highly physically active can *add* up to 3.5 years to your life. (Not smoking adds another 4.3.)

Having a *low* fitness level will not only kill you sooner, it is also more likely to leave you disabled and unable to live independently.

In fact, being more fit matters even if you have a higher BMI, because research shows that, at every level of BMI, fitter people live longer and are more likely to live independently than those who are physically unfit.

Among adults 65 and older, fitness is the single biggest discriminator between those who die sooner and those who live longer. In clinical studies, the highly fit have a death rate that is 60 percent lower than those who are unfit.

And it's almost never too late to increase your fitness. Research shows that men who increased their physical fitness level to highly fit during the 10 years between ages 50 and 60 eventually lowered their death rate by nearly one-third, compared to less fit individuals. The reduction in death rate achieved by improving fitness was as powerful as reducing smoking.

Constructing a science-driven lifestyle strategy does not *guarantee* long-term health success. It is, however, the most important tool for hedging your bets and adjusting the risk equation of life in your favor. The net effect of pursuing high fitness is that you are much more likely to have a trimmer waist, lower blood pressure, healthier blood lipids, less intravascular inflammation, and, consequently, a lower risk of heart disease and cancer, the top two causes of death.

Study after study demonstrates that lifestyle change centered on the pursuit of fitness is a life preserver that gives you the best possible opportunity to "die young at a very old age."

Exercising with a chronic condition. Maybe you've had a heart attack or stroke, or you have the intense breathlessness that accompanies chronic obstructive pulmonary disease (emphysema and/or chronic bronchitis), or you have low back pain.

"An adult with a chronic condition can obtain important health benefits from regular physical activity, but should be under the care of a health care provider," Dr. Neiman said.

More is merrier—and healthier. If you want "additional and more extensive health benefits," Dr. Neiman said that the PA Guidelines advise you to *double* your level of activity—to 300 minutes a week of moderate-intensity physical activity or 150 minutes a week of vigorous-intensity, or the equivalent combination.

Add muscle strengthening to the mix. The guidelines also advise adults to do moderate- to high-intensity muscle-strengthening activities, involving all major muscle groups (legs, hips, back, chest, abdomen, shoulders, and arms) on two or more days a week. "These activities provide additional health benefits," said Dr. Neiman.

Add the minutes you spend muscle strengthening to your weekly total of activity minutes.

How do you strengthen muscles? There are many ways.

You can lift weights. You can work out with resistance bands. You can do calisthenics—exercises that use your body for resistance, such as push-ups or sit-ups. You can work outside, if it involves strenuous activity, such as shoveling or moving rocks in a wheelbarrow. Even yoga is a very good activity for muscle strengthening.

Flexibility isn't recommended—but it can't hurt. "No specific recommendations for flexibility exercise were advanced," said Dr. Neiman. "But people are still encouraged to stretch because the increase in flexibility can allow people to more easily do activities that require greater flexibility.

Now you know what to do: it's easy, it's not particularly time-consuming—and it can save your life!

How to Start an Exercise Program

Here is advice for the best way to start—and stick with—an exercise program.

If you're starting an exercise program, exercise may seem downright intimidating. You look at all the people who are running, cycling, jazzercising, swimming, stair-stepping, and many of them don't look like they're having much fun. They sweating, panting—in fact, some of them look like they're dying!

It may seem odd to a nonexerciser, but these folks have chosen to do these activities because they *want* to do them. Maybe they love their new bodies. Maybe they love the camaraderie of their fellow exercisers. Maybe they like the challenge of a workout. Maybe they like the "high" exercise can give. Whatever the reason, they are exercising because they *like* to exercise.

And that's the most important point about exercise—you need to choose something you *like*. If you don't like your exercise routine, you'll do it for a few days and then quit. So maybe you find that you *really* like sitting on a stationary exercise bike—because you can read or watch the news at the same time you're getting fit. Maybe you find yoga rewarding, because it gives you an island of calm in a hectic day. We are confident that there is some form of exercise out there that you will enjoy. (Most people who exercise regularly end up choosing walking.) The trick is to find that exercise—and to have a place to do it that is easily accessible within your schedule.

Get Up and Sit-Up

One way to get your sit-ups in is to do them first thing in the morning.

Set your alarm to wake you up one minute earlier than usual. When your alarm goes off, roll onto your back and slide down a few inches until your heels catch on the mattress edge at the foot of the bed or your feet reach the footboard. Leave the covers on, put your hands behind your neck, and do a few sit-ups. Do them with your legs straight or bent, as you prefer. (You don't even have to open your eyes!)

Do as many as you can each morning. Even if you only manage one or two, that's better than none—and, if you keep with it, you'll soon be able to do more.

As discussed in this chapter, for optimal health and fitness, you need to find something you can do at least 21 to 22 minutes a day, for a total of 150 minutes a week. And you need to find a muscle-strengthening exercise you can do twice a week. The key is doing it *regularly*. If you walk twenty miles today and no miles at all for the rest of the month, your exercise is far from "regular." A moderate, 30-minute session at least five days a week is ideal. Remind yourself that the benefits of exercise are greatest when you exercise nearly every day.

If walking isn't for you, there are many other options—including some exotic ones. Consider tai chi, qi gong, or another martial art form. Consider a sport such as badminton or ping-pong. Consider outdoor activities such as gardening. Consider dancing.

Consider rebounding on a mini-trampoline—an exercise that requires only a single piece of equipment, and is incredibly convenient and easy. (Even if you hate exercise of all kinds, you should be willing to at least tolerate rebounding a few times a week.) Not only does rebounding increase heart rate like any other aerobic exercise, but it builds strength and is easy on the joints.

Remember, *any* exercise is fine—as long as it provides you with physical activity on a regular basis.

Start slowly

Many would-be exercisers charge into their new routine, and become quickly fatigued and discouraged. Whatever type of exercise you choose—start slowly. Exercise at a low intensity that you may not even feel at first *is* exercise—such as very slow walking—and stay with the activity for 10 or 20 minutes. By the end of the exercise session, you should feel some level of physical exertion, but you won't be exhausted. As the days go by, you will *naturally* find yourself wanting to increase your intensity level and the duration of exercise.

How to measure exercise intensity

A good way to figure out your intensity level is by using a measurement called your "target heart rate." To figure out your target heart rate, you first need to figure out your "maximum heart rate," the highest number of beats per minute (bpm) that is safe for your heart. To do that, subtract your age from 220. If you're 50, for example, your maximum heart rate is 170.

For moderate-intensity activity, you want your target heart rate at 50 to 70 percent of your maximum heart rate—or (in the case of our example) 85 to 119 beats per minute (bpm).

For vigorous-intensity physical activity, your heart rate should be 70 to 85 percent of your maximum heart rate. For our 50-year-old (who should be pretty fit by now!), that would be 119 to 144 bpm.

To determine whether or not you're exercising within your heart rate "target," you need to stop exercising briefly and take your pulse. The best place is the radial pulse, on the artery of the wrist in line with the thumb. Place the tips of your index and middle fingers over the artery and press lightly. (Don't use the thumb.) Starting the count on a beat, count for 60 seconds (timing your count with your watch), or count for 30 seconds and multiply by 2. If (continuing with the example of our 50-year-old friend) the number falls between 85 and 119, you're within the target heart rate for moderate-intensity physical activity.

Perceived exertion: another way to estimate intensity

We've described how to find your target heart rate using your pulse. There's another, and perhaps even simpler, way to measure your level of exercise

Ten Exercise Myths to Stop Believing

We asked David Neiman, PhD, Director of the Human Performance Lab at the North Carolina Research Campus, and author of *Exercise Testing and Prescription*, to debunk exercise myths that get in the way of maximizing the health power of physical activity. Here are his top 10, courtesy of the *Health and Fitness Journal* of the American College of Sports Medicine:

1. Exercise burns a lot of calories. Not really—in fact it's a lot fewer than you probably think. A brisk walk or jog of one mile burns about 90 to 110 calories. Thirty minutes of moderate- to vigorous-intensity exercise burns 200 to 400 calories—the amount found in a bagel! There are many benefits from physical activity, but weight-loss isn't really one of them.

2. Sit-ups are a good way to reduce belly fat. Consider this fact: a pound of human fat contains 3,500 calories. Sit-ups burn three to five calories *per minute* (and most people can't go beyond one minute). Do the math: it would take more than 10 hours of sit-ups to burn one pound of fat! A regular program of abdominal exercises will tighten the muscles and reduce your waistline, but the layer of fat over the muscles will remain—unless you burn more calories than you take in.

3. After exercise, your metabolism is revved up all day, **burning many extra calories.** Sorry, it's a myth! The truth is that after 30 to 45 minutes of vigorous exercise, the body's metabolism quickly returns to pre-exercise levels, and only 10 to 25 extra calories are burned (the amount in a bite of apple). Another way to look at it: if you're overweight and you take a 20- to 30-minute walk, you'll burn 10 extra calories afterward.

4. Just 15 minutes of aerobic exercise, three days a week, is **enough to promote health.** This is a recommendation from the 1960s, and it has *not* stood the test of time. We now know the body needs a lot more exercise. The current and best recommendation are the Physical Activity Guidelines (discussed in this chapter)—anywhere from 75 to 150 minutes a week, depending on the intensity. But the good news is that you can get that exercise in sessions of as little as 10 minutes, and still derive all the health benefits.

5. Aerobic fitness is a lot more important than muscular **fitness for health.** This is another myth from the 1960s. Brisk walking, jogging, or cycling is *not* enough for good health. You also need muscle-strengthening exercises (as discussed in this chapter). Strong muscles are a must for strong bones and preventing osteoporosis. And the American Heart Association (AHA)—which has long recommended heart-strengthening aerobic activity—now also recommends muscle strengthening. "The potential benefits, not only to cardiovascular health but also to weight management and the prevention of disability and falls, are becoming more widely appreciated," says a statement from the AHA.

6. Exercise depletes the body of many vitamins and **minerals, so use supplements to stay in balance.** If you eat enough high-quality food, you don't need supplements to support an exercise program. However, some nutritional deficiencies, such as iron, can impair your ability to exercise.

7. Stretch before you exercise. Stretching is more effective when your muscles are *already* warm. So it's far better to stretch *after* exercise than before. And stretching has turned out to be of far less value to health than originally claimed. When is stretching important? For athletic performance, and during rehabilitation from joint injuries. But there's little need to place much emphasis on stretching in your exercise routine—for health, or for injury prevention.

8. The best time to exercise is in the morning. Good news for night owls who have a hard time waking up in the morning: the benefits of exercise are the same no matter when you exercise—morning, afternoon, or evening. In a study Dr. Neiman conducted, half the participants exercised in the morning and the other half in the afternoon—and the benefits of exercise for fitness, and the decrease of risk factors for disease and psychological health, were the same in both groups. Choose a time of day that works best for you—the time when you enjoy exercise the most, and will do it regularly.

9. Individuals who regularly exercise need less sleep than their sedentary peers. The truth is just the opposite: people who exercise tend to need *more* sleep to restore their well-used muscles. In fact, a study shows that people who exercise regularly fall asleep faster and sleep longer and deeper than people who don't exercise.

10. You need to join a health/fitness club or enlist the services of a personal trainer to be fit. Not true. The best motivation for long-term exercise comes from within. If you need a health/fitness club or personal trainer to stay motivated—great. If you don't, no problem. The best fitness solution: find an exercise that works for you and a routine that fits into your schedule—and let that routine becomes as regular and necessary as eating and sleeping.

intensity, and that's the technique called *perceived exertion*—how hard you *feel* your body is working, based on the sensations you experience during physical activity: a faster heart rate, faster breathing, sweating, and tired muscles. Studies show it's a pretty accurate way of estimating your intensity level.

The scale that is typically used for perceived exertion is the "Borg Scale," which ranges from 6 to 20, with 6 being no exertion at all and 20 being maximal exertion. Here's the scale:

7: Extremely light
9: Very light (like walking slowly for several minutes)
11: Light
13: Somewhat hard (moderate intensity; it feels okay to continue)
15: Hard (vigorous intensity)
17: Very hard (vigorous intensity; you can go on, but you really have to push yourself, and you're tired)
19: Extremely hard (vigorous intensity; the most strenuous activity you've ever experienced)

"When exercising at the 'somewhat hard' level, you can think, talk intermittently with a partner, look around and enjoy the scenery, and engage in prolonged endurance activity," Dr. Neiman told us.

"When exercising at the 'very hard' level, the pulse is too high, and it is difficult to exercise for prolonged periods of time," he continued.

"When exercising below 'somewhat hard,' the exercise won't strengthen your heart and lungs."

Now you know that exercise generates NO . . . NO protects the heart . . . all you need is 22 minutes a day of exercise at a moderate level of intensity . . . and how to measure your intensity level. Time to get started!

FIVE

NO-How: More Smart Methods to Increase NO

From Naps to Saunas, Increasing NO Is a Gas!

Diet, supplements, and exercise aren't the only way to boost NO in your body. Far from it.

There are *many* easy-to-do actions that you can take to increase your body's production of NO.

And just as with eating more NO-enhancing foods and taking NO-enhancing supplements, these simple strategies can help you *prevent* or *reverse* the many diseases linked to low NO, such as high blood pressure, heart disease, and stroke—the diseases that kill the majority of Americans.

Now, most of these additional NO-boosting strategies aren't all that surprising (though one or two are). After all, how many times have you been told by stress experts to breathe deeply . . . by exercise experts to exercise regularly . . . by nutritionists to drink more water. What is surprising, however, is that now we understand one of the main reasons *why* these oft-repeated health suggestions *work*—because they increase NO!

Let's take a look at these additional NO-boosting strategies one by one.

Breathe Deeply: The Nose NOs

Breathing is pretty, well, *basic*.

You can stop eating for a couple of weeks and stay alive. You can stop drinking water and survive for a few days. But stop breathing—and you'll be dead in a matter of minutes. The obvious reason: your body requires oxygen to work, and it requires it *now*.

"To breathe is to live," is how Dennis Lewis, author of *The Tao of Natural*

Breathing, summed up the situation for us. "To breathe *fully* is to live *fully*," he added. However, he went on, few of us *actually* breathe fully. And maybe that's why we're gasping for good health.

"Our chronic shallow breathing reduces the working capacity of our respiratory system to only about one-third of its potential," said Lewis. "Shallow breathing diminishes the exchange of gases, and thus the production of energy in our cells. It deprives us of the many healthful actions that breathing naturally would have on our inner organs. It cuts us off from our real feelings. Shallow breathing promotes disharmony and 'dis-ease' at every level of our lives." (If you feel tense after reading that description of all the bad things that shallow breathing can do to you—take a calming deep breath!)

Science provides support for many of Lewis's statements.

Lowering high blood pressure

For example, research shows that regular practice of slow, deep breathing—10 to 15 minutes a day, for three to four weeks—can lower blood pressure (hypertension).

In one study, Israeli researchers conducted an experiment with 17 people who had "resistant" hypertension—high blood pressure that isn't lowered by medications. They put all the hypertensives on a daily regimen of 15 minutes of slow, deep breathing, using a device called RESPeRATE. After eight weeks, 14 of the 17 hypertensives had responded to deep breathing. The average drop in blood pressure measured in the doctor's office was 12.9 systolic and 6.9 diastolic, and the average drop measured at home was 6.4 systolic and 2.6 diastolic—a *very* significant decrease in blood pressure. (Measurements of blood pressure at the doctor's office are typically higher, because most people are somewhat anxious at the doctor's, a phenomenon called white coat hypertension.)

In a similar study, 66 people with type 2 diabetes and hypertension were divided into two groups: 33 practiced slow, deep breathing and 33 didn't. After eight weeks, those practicing deep breathing had a drop of blood pressure of 10.0 systolic and 3.6 diastolic; there was no change among those in the other group.

The results were published in the *Journal of Human Hypertension*.

Deeper breathing, better health

Lower blood pressure is only one benefit from deeper, slower breathing; there are many others.

Anxiety. A regimen including deep breathing decreased anxiety levels by 57 percent, report physicians at the Canadian College of Naturopathic Medicine in Toronto.

Arrhythmia. Although often harmless, these irregular heart rhythms can increase the risk of a heart attack if you have heart disease. In a study in the *International Journal of Cardiology*, doctors reported that slow, deep breathing reduces one type of arrhythmia (premature ventricular contractions [PVCs] , or "skipped beats") by at least 50 percent.

Asthma. Asthma patients who received training in deep breathing had milder symptoms of asthma and reduced their need for medications, reported a team of Canadian researchers in the journal *Archives of Physical Medicine and Rehabilitation*. And in a study in the medical journal *The Lancet*, asthma patients who were taught slow, deep breathing had stronger lungs, fewer symptoms, and used less asthma medication.

Heart attacks. Researchers in Korea studied 58 people with heart disease who had undergone an angiography (a surgical procedure to unblock and widen a clogged artery). Thirty received instruction in stress management, including deep breathing; 28 didn't. Those who learned deep breathing had fewer heart attacks, lower artery-clogging LDL cholesterol, and better overall "quality of life."

In another study, Dutch researchers added deep breathing to the cardiac rehabilitation program of people who had suffered a heart attack. Those who received the training had fewer arrhythmias and a lower resting heart rate (a sign of a stronger heart), compared to people in the program who didn't.

Researchers in Sweden studied 90 people after coronary bypass surgery, teaching 48 of them deep-breathing. Those who learned and practiced the technique had much less atelectasis, or collapse of the lung (a common side effect of this surgery). And 72 percent of those who learned deep breathing said they thought it helped them. The findings were in the medical journal *Chest*.

Low back pain. Canadian researchers studied 75 people with chronic low back pain, providing 39 of them with non-drug treatments that included deep breathing. After three months, the deep breathing group had 62 percent less back pain. The breathing group also had a much better mental outlook (not surprisingly, since they were in less pain), more spinal flexibility—and even lost more weight!

Smoking cessation. A study in the journal *Addictive Behaviors* reported that deep breathing decreased withdrawal symptoms in people trying to quit smoking: craving for cigarettes, irritability, and tension.

Why is deep breathing so effective in blowing away bad health?

For one thing, shallow breathing makes the blood more acidic. (Your body is constantly maintaining a balance between two types of basic chemical compounds—acids and alkalis—in order to keep your body fluids slightly alkaline.) Acidic blood makes the kidneys less efficient at removing sodium from the blood—and that extra sodium can trigger high blood pressure.

For another, slow, deep breathing activates the parasympathetic nervous system, the part of our nervous system that allows us to calm down and relax after stress—and excess stress plays a role in dozens of conditions and diseases, from colds to heart disease.

But here's what most people don't know about deep breathing: it increases NO.

The highest concentrations of NO in the body are found in the *nasal passages*, in the back of the nose. When you breathe deeply through your nose, your transport NO to your lungs. That extra NO opens up the lungs, allowing you to absorb more oxygen and expel more carbon dioxide. (It's a small but very impactful 3 percent increase.) And because this is an NO-mediated effect, breathing through the NO-rich nose makes all the difference in the positive effects: researchers found that nose breathing led to a 10 to 15 percent higher oxidation of the blood than mouth breathing. That's right: the same amount of breath—but much more oxidation, because of NO.

How to breathe deeply

To find out the best way to breathe deeply, we talked with Fred Luskin, PhD, an associate professor at the Institute of Transpersonal Psychology in Palo Alto, California, and coauthor of *Stress Free for Good*. "The simplest and most direct form of stress management is to change your shallow, stressed breathing into belly breathing," he told us.

Here are his six-step instructions. (Remember: to make sure deep breathing is NO-producing, follow these instructions inhaling and exhaling *through your nose*.)

1. As you inhale, imagine that your belly is a big balloon that you're slowly filling with air.
2. Place your hands on your belly while you slowly inhale.
3. Watch your hands as they rise with your in-breath.
4. Watch your hands fall as you slowly breathe out, letting the air out of the balloon.
5. As you exhale, make sure your belly stays relaxed.
6. Take at least two or three more slow and deep breaths, making sure to keep your attention on the rise and fall of your belly.

"Make sure you practice every single day," said Dr. Luskin. "For example," he said, "breathe deeply when you're sitting in your car, watching TV, walking for exercise, or sitting at the computer at work."

He advises you to sometimes breathe deeply for as long as 5 to 10 minutes—and we heartily (and lungily) agree with that advice!

H$_2$O and NO: Hydrate Your Way to Health

Let's cut right to the chase: not drinking enough water every day reduces the activity of nitric oxide synthase (NOS), enzymes that help convert L-arginine to NO.

And that reduction of NO might be the reason why a study from researchers at the Loma Linda University School of Public Health produced these remarkable findings about water and heart disease:

- Women who drank five or more glasses of water a day had a 59 percent lower risk of dying from heart disease, compared to women who drank two or fewer glasses.

- Men who drink five or more glasses of water a day had a 46 percent lower risk of dying from heart disease, compared to men who drank two or fewer glasses.

That's the same level of protection provided by exercising regularly, lowering cholesterol, or quitting smoking!

The lead researcher of the study, Jacqueline Chan, PhD, an assistant professor of public health at Loma Linda University, told us that other research shows drinking plenty of water every day can:

- prevent colon cancer, the #2 cancer in America.
- satisfy appetite during dieting, so you shed more pounds.
- soothe the aching joints of arthritis.
- stop a recurrence of kidney stones.
- reduce the incidence of bladder infections, a chronic problem for millions of American women.
- cut the number and severity of asthma attacks.
- help prevent complications from diabetes.
- boost the immune system, thereby providing extra protection against a wide range of serious and everyday conditions.
- rev up your physical and mental performance, for more energy, a better memory, and improved concentration.

Other experts we talked with added to the list of water's many preventive and curative benefits:

Cataracts. Drinking plenty of water can help prevent cataracts, said Marc Grossman, OD, LAc, an optometrist in private practice in Rye and New Paltz, New York, and medical director of the website www.naturaleye care.com. "Drinking eight to ten, eight-ounce glasses a day maintains the flow of nutrients to the lens and the release of waste and toxins from the tissues."

Chapped lips. "Chapped lips are often the first sign of not drinking enough water," said Victoria Nash, an esthetician in Phoenix, Arizona, and founder of the skin care company Esenté Physioceuticals. "In fact, I can tell if someone hasn't been drinking enough water simply by looking at their lips—they're always dry and cracked."

Constipation. "Getting enough water is the number one action to counter constipation," said Stella Metsovas, CN, a nutritionist in Laguna Beach, California. "If you're dehydrated—and many people are—it's more likely your stool will be hard, dry, and difficult to pass."

Dry eyes. "Water is needed by all the organs in the body—including the eyes," said Robert Latkany, MD, founder and director of the Dry Eye Clinic at the New York Eye and Ear Infirmary, and author of *The Dry Eye Remedy*.

Kidney stones. To *prevent* a kidney stone, drink 60 to 80 ounces of water a day, recommended Bryan Kansas, MD, a urologist in Austin, Texas. "People think they're drowning themselves in fluid—but most people aren't even drinking 40 ounces a day," he said. If you've already had one or more kidney stones, he advised drinking 128 ounces a day (16 eight-ounce glasses) to prevent a recurrence.

Repetitive strain injury (RSI). "To reduce the pain of RSI, such as carpal tunnel, stay well-hydrated," said Robert E. Markison, MD, a hand surgeon in San Francisco. "It delivers pain-relieving oxygen and nutrients into the areas hit by RSI."

Ulcer pain. "If you drink four to six glasses during an episode of ulcer pain, the pain may disappear," said Liz Lipski, PhD, CCN, a certified clinical nutritionist in Ashville, North Carolina, and author of *Digestive Wellness*.

Urinary tract infections (UTI). To stop recurrent UTIs, drink at least one-half your body weight in ounces of water every day—for example, if you weight 140 pounds, drink at least 70 ounces, said Holly Lucille, ND, a naturopathic physician in private practice in Los Angeles.

Why water works

Water does more than deliver extra NO to your cells, of course.

"Without water, nothing lives," wrote F. Batmanghelidj, MD, in his book *Water for Health, for Healing, for Life*. He enumerates the many reasons why your body needs water every day. Health-giving H_2O:

- generates electrical and magnetic energy in every cell.
- provides the "bonding adhesive" in cellular architecture.

- prevents DNA damage and helps repair DNA.
- increases the efficiency of the immune system.
- acts as the main solvent for the breakdown of food into nutrients.
- transports all substances in the body.
- maintains the volume of the blood.
- increases the efficiency of red blood cells in collecting oxygen in the lungs.
- brings oxygen to the cells and removes waste gases.
- helps manufacture neurotransmitters, the messenger molecules that relay messages from neuron to neuron in your brain.

We'll add a very important item to that list in a country where just about everybody complains about feeling tired a lot of the time: water helps keep energy levels stable. In fact, some studies show that poor hydration is the #1 cause of daytime fatigue! Try drinking a glass or two of water the next time you feel tired—you'll be amazed at how quickly you perk up!

And if you're like most Americans, you *don't* drink the 8 to 10, eight-ounce glasses of water every day that is necessary to keep your system lubricated. (Recommendations vary, but that's the amount we think is best for health.)

Instead, we Americans drink coffee, tea, soda, juices, and energy drinks. And while these fluids might temporarily quench your thirst, they are *not* a replacement for water.

Defeating dehydration
Are you dehydrated?

Thirst is the most obvious sign, of course—although by the time you're really thirsty, your body is parched!

Natural-minded doctor Jacob Teitelbaum, MD, author of *From Fatigued to Fantastic*, told us there's a very easy way to tell: if your lips are dry, you're dry inside, too! Other signs of mild dehydration include chronic pain in joints and muscles, low back pain, headaches, and constipation. Also, your urine might have a strong odor, with a yellow or amber (rather than clear) color.

To make sure you have all the water you need, keep a bottle of water handy whenever you're working, traveling, or exercising. If you become bored with plain water, add a bit of lemon or lime.

A couple of addition tips:

- Alcohol is dehydrating; if you drink alcohol, drink more water.
- Sodas *aren't* a replacement for water—and deliver way too many calories.
- Noncaffeinated herbal teas can count toward water consumption. But caffeinated teas (and coffee) are diuretics: they drain the body of more fluid than they put in.
- Sports drinks with electrolytes are often good fluid replacements—but they also contain a lot of sugar and calories that you don't need, and studies show they're also rough on your teeth, stripping enamel.

Tossing and Turning Off NO

There's a lot of intriguing (though not definitive) evidence about NO and sleep, showing that (1) low NO may cause insomnia, and (2) insomnia lowers NO. (Medical experts call this kind of relationship *bidirectional*: Factor A makes Factor B worse, which further worsens Factor A. Another example from the world of sleep: heartburn worsens insomnia, and the insomnia further worsens heartburn.)

But whatever the relationship between NO and sleep, one thing is for sure: a *lot* of us are poor sleepers.

Chronic insomnia is defined as having trouble falling asleep or staying asleep, or waking up too early, at least three times a month—and an estimated 45 million Americans fit that definition. Sixty million of us have those same symptoms, but less often. That's 100 million American insomniacs!

Insomnia causes daytime fatigue, of course, and that's bad enough—a study shows that people with insomnia have 32 percent more absenteeism,

70 percent more reduced productivity, and 49 percent more accidents at work.

But too little sleep also causes *disease.*

Studies show that insomnia can cause or contribute to:

Mortality. Yes, *death.* People who slept less than six hours a night had up to a five times higher death rate than people who slept more.

Anxiety. Insomniacs were six times more likely to suffer from "generalized anxiety disorder" (GAD)—near-constant worrying that interferes with your ability to function day-to-day.

Burnout. Insomniacs were 64 percent more likely to suffer from exhaustion caused by long-term stress.

Depression. Insomniacs were 42 percent more likely to be depressed, found Dutch researchers.

Diabetes. Insomniacs had nearly three times the risk of developing type 2 diabetes.

Heartburn. Insomnia tripled the risk for heartburn.

Overweight. In a seven-year study, people who had trouble falling asleep were 65 percent more likely to have major weight gain.

Chronic pain. Insomniacs had three times the risk of having chronic pain.

Of course, if insomnia lowers NO, you'd expect a link between insomnia and high blood pressure, heart disease, and stroke. And that link definitely exists:

High blood pressure. Poor sleepers were 32 percent more likely to have high blood pressure. And people who slept five hours or less a night were five times more likely to have high blood pressure.

Heart disease. People who slept less than seven to eight hours a night had *double* the risk of dying from a heart attack, found UK researchers.

Stroke. People who slept six or fewer hours a night were 22 percent more likely to suffer a stroke.

Evidence linking insomnia and low NO

Here's a sampling of some of the most recent scientific evidence—from studies on laboratory animals and people—linking poor sleep and NO.

Circadian rhythms—NO plays a role. Circadian rhythms—the body's sleep-wake cycle, in response to light—are controlled by a "clock" in the brain called the suprachiasmatic nucleus (SCN). In a paper in the journal *Reviews in Endocrine and Metabolic Disorders*, researchers at the University of Calgary discuss how "light information" is relayed via the eye to the brain—and theorize that NO may play a role.

Insomniac mice have low NO. Noting that "NO is thought to be involved in the regulation of both sleep and circadian rhythms," researchers in Switzerland studied mice bred to be deficient in cGMP, a signaling compound activated by NO. They found the mice had odd sleep patterns, less REM sleep, and more wakefulness.

NO helps mice recover from sleep deprivation. Researchers in India found that a drug that reversed the effects of sleep deprivation in mice (anxiety-like behavior, impairment in movement, and cellular damage) worked because it boosted NO levels. The findings were in the journal *Behavioural Brain Research*.

Are age-related sleep problems caused by low NO? Sleep worsens with age: 58 percent of adults age 59 and over report having difficulty sleeping at least a few nights a week. Finnish researchers measured NO levels in young (four months), middle-aged (14 months), and old (24 months) rats. They found that, compared to young rats, old rats' NO didn't increase in the brain during sleep deprivation, and that infusing the old animals with NO didn't induce sleep. "These results support our hypothesis that aging impairs the mechanism through which NO in the [brain] induces sleep," concluded the researchers, in *Neurobiology of Aging*.

More NO during dreaming. In a study of patients with memory loss and Alzheimer's, researchers in Taiwan found that neuronal nitric oxide synthase (nNOS)—the enzyme that triggers the production of NO—is increased during rapid eye movement (REM) sleep, the period of time when we dream. The results were in the *Journal of Clinical Neuroscience*.

NO and sleep apnea. In obstructive sleep apnea (OSA), you're roused to semiconsciousness repeatedly during the night because sagging soft tissue at the back of the throat plugs your airway. It afflicts an estimated 30 million Americans, many of them overweight men. And it dramatically increases the risk for heart disease and stroke. Is there a connection between NO, sleep apnea, and heart disease?

Highly likely, said French researchers, writing in the *American Journal of Pathology*, in August 2010. They studied 62 people with OSA and found that many had reduced NO production and impaired endothelial function—and they theorized that it's low NO that might cause the arterial disease so common in people with OSA.

In a similar study, researchers at the Sleep Heart Program at Ohio State University found that men with OSA had 40 percent poorer endothelial function than men without the disease. The results were in the *American Journal of Respiratory and Critical Care Medicine*.

And researchers at the Columbia University College of Physicians and Surgeons studied 71 people, including 38 with untreated OSA. They found eNOS levels and endothelial function were much lower in people with OSA—and when those folks were treated for sleep apnea, their eNOS levels and endothelial function improved. The results were in the medical journal *Circulation*.

How to get a great night's sleep

All these studies point to what is probably the fact of the matter: NO plays a key role in sleep, and poor sleep lowers NO.

Here are Dr. Zand's recommendations for a better night's sleep. Try one or more:

Watch out for caffeine close to bedtime. Don't ingest any foods or drinks containing caffeine too close to bedtime. A caffeine "buzz" lasts for six to eight hours, so time your last coffee, tea, or chocolate accordingly.

Ditto for alcohol. Don't drink alcohol within two hours of going to bed—it causes light sleep, and as the effect wears off you might find yourself waking up in the middle of the night.

Don't exercise right before bed. Leave at least three hours between when you workout and conk out.

Eat tryptophan-containing foods. Tryptophan is an amino acid the brain uses to make serotonin, a brain chemical that regulates sleep. High tryptophan foods include bananas, cottage cheese, fish, dates, milk, peanuts, and turkey.

Take these sleep-inducing supplements. A muscle-relaxing magnesium-calcium supplement, with 500 milligrams (mg) of calcium and 250 mg of magnesium, can help if you experience sleeplessness accompanied by leg cramps.

Melatonin is a hormone vital to the sleep-wake cycle, and is often low in seniors. Try 3 mg one-half hour to two hours before retiring.

A balanced multivitamin-mineral supplement can also help.

Chamomile tea. Prepare and drink a cup of this relaxing tea an hour before bedtime.

Sniff some lavender oil. This aromatherapy scent can help usher insomniacs into dreamland. Add a few drops to your hot bath, inhale directly from the bottle, or diffuse lavender into your bedroom air. You can also put a drop or two in a spray bottle full of distilled water, shake gently, and spray the mixture on your pillow shortly before bed.

"Sleep hygiene"—the daily habits that help you sleep—are crucially important. They include:

Set a sleep schedule and stick to it. Establishing and keeping a set time for going to bed and rising in the morning is one of the best ways to prevent and cure insomnia.

Relax before bedtime. Follow a simple regimen to slow down your metabolic rate and unwind before retiring. Sip a cup of herbal tea, read something light, listen to soothing music, or practice a relaxation technique, such as deep breathing.

Take a hot bath. Soaking in a hot bath for thirty minutes before bed can help you fall asleep faster, experience less wakefulness during the night, and awaken feeling refreshed. Best: allow two hours between the bath and going to bed, because a high body temperature can keep you awake.

Keep your bedroom quiet, dark, and cool. Studies show that's the right environment for deep, restful sleep.

Bacteria, NO, and the Curse of Ultra-Cleanliness

Consider this scientific fact: there are more bacteria living on and in your body than there are cells in your body—about 100 trillion bacteria, 10 times the number of cells.

Are they hanging out waiting for the perfect opportunity to infect you?

Absolutely not. Believe it or not, most of those bacteria are there to *help* you. They're "good" or "friendly" bacteria that play a supporting role in keeping you healthy.

For example, the good bacteria in your colon play many roles. They keep bad bacteria and disease-causing fungi in check, produce B-vitamins and vitamin K, aid in the absorption of nutrients such as magnesium and calcium, manufacture natural antibiotics and boost the production of immune cells, break down and rebuild hormones, and even kill cancer cells. See—those bacteria are *very* friendly!

And good bacteria also play a key role in producing NO.

On your skin, *ammonia-oxidizing bacteria* change ammonia into nitrate and then into nitrite, at which point your naturally acidic sweat causes the nitrite to form NO—which fights off disease-causing bacteria and fungal infections.

In your mouth, bacteria (mostly residing in the tongue) also transform nitrate in food into nitrite, and in the stomach the nitrite is transformed to NO. Without the bacteria, you don't get any NO from the foods you eat!

In your gut, friendly bacteria reduce nitrate and nitrite to NO.

But most of us seem to think bacteria—all bacteria—need to be wiped out. There are now more than 700 antibacterial products on the market, up from just a few dozen in the 1990s. There are antibacterial soaps, hand lotions, and toothbrushes; antibacterial cleansers, dishwashing detergents, and window cleaners; antibacterial pillows, sheets, towels, and slippers— there are even antibacterial chopsticks!

In a presentation titled "Antibacterial Products: A Cause For Concern," Stuart B. Levy, MD—professor of molecular biology and microbiology and of medicine at Tufts University School of Medicine—criticized this "antibacterial craze."

"We exist in the bacterial world, not bacteria in ours," said Dr. Levy. "Unfortunately, we believe that we can rid ourselves of bacteria when, in fact, we cannot. Instead, we should 'make peace' with them. Although we need to control pathogens when they cause disease, we do not have to engage in a full-fledged 'war' against the microbial world."

And that full-fledged war has unexpected collateral damage—it destroys NO!

A little dirt is good for you

Here are some suggestions for reducing your use of antibacterial products to maintain the optimal levels of good NO-producing bacteria:

Don't be afraid to get outside and get dirty. This replenishes the NO-creating bacteria on your skin.

Don't bathe more than once a day. It's even okay to go a day without taking a bath!

Only use antibiotics when absolutely necessary. The more antibiotics that you and others take, the more bacteria mutate to develop resistance to them—"bad" bacteria that can also kill the good NO-generating bacteria. Case in point: every year 18 million Americans are prescribed antibiotics for acute sinus infections. But studies show antibiotics don't work for this problem—they don't lessen the severity of symptoms or shorten the bout of sinusitis. "Antibiotics are not justified for acute sinusitis," said a team of doctors reporting in the medical journal *The Lancet.*

Don't use antibacterial hand soap. Hand-washing with regular soap is adequate.

Don't use antibacterial mouthwash. Research shows that the use of antibacterial mouthwash *drastically* reduces levels of NO in the stomach. Brushing your teeth twice a day is plenty of protection from gum disease and decay.

Saunas: NO Is Hot!

A sauna is a small area where you're exposed to intensified dry or wet heat, usually from 160 to 180°F.

The research showing that saunas can boost NO has an international pedigree: it began in Japan, with a study using Syrian golden hamsters.

Noting that saunas improve endothelial function and symptoms in patients with congestive heart failure, or CHF (a heart permanently weakened by a heart attack, severe high blood pressure, or other heart-damaging cause), Japanese researchers wondered whether the saunas worked by increasing nitric oxide synthase (eNOS), the enzyme that triggers the production of NO.

To find out, they put one group of hamsters in a sauna for 20 minutes a day for one month. (The study didn't say whether the hamsters also received a massage, a facial, or any other spa services.) A "control" group of hamsters didn't receive sauna therapy.

After four weeks, the scientists found the sauna hamsters had 50 percent higher arterial levels of eNOS than the non-sauna hamsters. After the first week, the sauna hamsters also had a 40 times greater level of genetic materials that trigger the production of eNOS.

"Repeated thermal [sauna] therapy upregulates eNOS expression in arterial endothelium," concluded the researchers in the *Japanese Circulation Journal*.

In their next study, published four years later in 2005, the researchers once again conducted an experiment on sauna therapy and eNOS—but this time in hamsters with experimentally induced CHF. The researchers found that four weeks of sauna therapy significantly increased the genetic expression of eNOS in the arteries of the CHF hamsters, and increased nitrate concentrations in the blood. CHF hamsters that didn't undergo sauna therapy showed no change.

"Repeated sauna therapy increases eNOS expression and NO production in hamsters with heart failure," concluded the researchers.

A year later, the same team of researchers found that sauna therapy improved the growth of new blood vessels (angiogenesis) in mice—and did so because of the increase of eNOS.

All well and good—but can saunas actually *treat* cardiovascular disease in humans? Several studies show the answer is yes.

In a study in the *Journal of the American College of Cardiology*, a team of researchers found that sauna therapy improved peripheral arterial disease (PAD)—severe blockages in the arteries of the legs, causing pain during walking and hard-to-heal leg ulcers.

In a paper in the July 2009 issue of the journal *Medical Hypotheses*, scientists noted that sauna therapy boosts eNOS to levels similar to that from exercise (which we talk about in Chapter 4), and that sauna therapy might be a way to boost NO in people "too physically impaired for significant aerobic activity." They also noted that if you don't have a sauna, "regular hot baths at home may suffice as practical thermal therapy."

Take a Probiotic

"Probiotic" is a word meaning both the friendly bacteria in the gut or a nutritional supplement containing those friendly bacteria. And scientific studies show those probiotic supplements can help prevent and treat a wide variety of conditions, including:

- eczema and other allergy-caused skin problems
- inflammatory bowel disease (IBD)
- irritable bowel syndrome (IBS)
- diverticular disease (inflammation of pouches in the intestinal tract)
- diarrhea
- lactose intolerance
- indigestion
- flatulence
- antibiotic side effects
- anxiety in fibromyalgia and chronic fatigue syndrome (gut bacteria help generate brain-balancing neurochemicals)
- vaginal infections
- respiratory infections (colds, flu, pneumonia)

And in a paper in the April 2010 issue of *Circulation Journal* (the journal of the Japanese Circulation Society), the researchers who have conducted most of the eNOS/sauna research to date summarized their findings.

The ideal NO-boosting sauna

First, they said they found that the best type of sauna to use to boost NO is an infrared sauna (which warms up the sauna without the need for moisture, so the air is warm and dry, as compared to the humid air found in traditional saunas). They also recommended the temperature stay at 140°F, lower than the typical sauna. You stay in the sauna for 15 minutes, and then rest outside the sauna, laying down for 30 minutes, while covered in blankets.

You drink water during the process so you don't become dehydrated.

- gum disease (gingivitis)
- rheumatoid arthritis
- pancreatitis (inflammation or infection of the pancreas, the organ that helps control blood sugar)
- colon cancer

Big list—and it's not even complete! That's why it's smart to take a probiotic supplement to stay in good health or restore good health. But it's also smart to take one to ensure the production of NO.

Two studies from the world-famous Karolinska Institute in Sweden showed that the friendly bacteria *Lactobacilli* and *Bifidobacteria* generated NO from nitrite (whereas unfriendly bacteria such as *Escherichia coli* and *Clostridium difficile* did *not* generate NO).

"We conclude that NO can be generated by the . . . gut flora [friendly bacteria] in the presence of nitrate or nitrite," concluded the researchers in the medical journal *Nitric Oxide*. And in a subsequent scientific paper, the researchers speculated that probiotic bacteria in the gut may generate "beneficial effects" *because* they generate NO.

They call this particular type of sauna "Waon therapy," meaning "soothing warmth" therapy.

They have found the therapy lessens the severity of CHF (decreasing the rate of hospitalization and death), and point out that the therapy increases endothelial function—a sure sign of increased NO.

"We believe that eNOS upregulation induced by repeated Waon therapy is caused by an increase in cardiac output and blood flow . . . although thermal stimulation might alternatively upregulate arterial eNOS directly." In other words, the effect is exercise-like, stimulating circulation, or it might be the heat itself that does it.

They also noted that Waon therapy improves PAD, decreasing pain and speeding the healing of leg ulcers. And they have also used the therapy to treat high blood pressure, high cholesterol, diabetes, and obesity.

"An ideal therapy for the 21st century should be safe, free of side effects, and have high medical value (ie, high benefit/cost ratio)," concluded the researchers. "It should be non-invasive and make patients feel better. Waon therapy fulfills all these criteria and is therefore a promising therapy for patients with cardiovascular diseases such as CHF and PAD."

We couldn't agree more—particularly because the therapy works by naturally boosting NO! In fact, we think maybe they should start calling it a SauNO rather than a sauna . . .

Resource: You can find an excellent company that sells infrared saunas—High Tech Health—on the web at www.hightechhealth.com.

Chant OM, Increase NO

In a scientific paper in the *International Journal of Molecular Medicine*, titled "Examination of Meditation's Therapeutic and Global Medicinal Outcomes Via Nitric Oxide," researchers in the Neuroscience Research Institute at the State University of New York theorized that relaxation techniques work to improve so many different health problems—high blood pressure, heart arrhythmias, chronic pain, insomnia, anxiety, depression, PMS, and infertility—because they increase NO, which has a "global healing effect."

We couldn't agree more with their hypothesis!

Here is an effective relaxation technique that you can practice to help you increase NO.

The "One" Relaxation Technique
1. Sit or lie quietly in a comfortable position.
2. To minimize distraction, close your eyes.
3. Consciously relax all of your muscles, beginning at your feet and progressing upward to your face. To practice "letting go," give a good shake and then relax.
4. Breathe through your nose easily and naturally. On each outgoing breath, say the word *one* silently to yourself. Concentrating on the word *one* helps keep intrusive thoughts away.

5. Once your muscles are relaxed, continue breathing easily and regularly for 10 to 15 minutes. Sit or lie quietly for several more minutes after you are finished, at first with your eyes closed, then with your eyes open.

If you don't achieve a deep level of relaxation, don't worry.

Try to maintain a passive attitude. Relaxation will happen at its own pace. Distracting thoughts will vanish as long as you don't dwell on them. Silently repeating the word *one* helps. With practice, the relaxation response will come with little effort.

This technique can be practiced during the day, but it is the most helpful just before bedtime. Because digestion can interfere with the relaxation response, the exercise should not be practiced for two hours after eating.

The "Tense to Relax" Relaxation Technique

A somewhat similar relaxation technique, offered to us by Dr. Luskin, is a method he calls "Tense to Relax." Here's how to do it:

1. Take two slow, deep belly breaths. (See the section "How to breathe deeply" on page 114 for complete instructions on how to belly breathe.)
2. On the third inhalation, tighten your right arm from your shoulder to your hand.
3. Hold tightly for two or three seconds.
4. As you exhale, relax fully and let your arm drop.
5. Repeat the first four steps with your other arm, each leg, and then your entire body.
6. As you practice, repeat a relaxing affirmation, such as "I have all the time in the world," or "I am relaxed and at peace."

"When you tense your muscles in this technique, *really* tense them," he advised. "When you relax, *really* relax. And remember that you're capable of this kind of relaxation at *any* time."

And Dr. Luskin recommends *doing* the technique any time, but particularly to feel alert when you first wake up in the morning, when you're sitting at your desk, when you're stuck in traffic, when you're sitting in an airplane, before physical exercise, when your neck and shoulders are tight, and before going to bed.

Traditional Chinese Medicine: The Ancient Way of NO

Western medicine—the medicine of high-tech diagnosis, targeted pharmaceuticals, and surgery—has been a miracle for humankind. For example:

Vaccines have brought smallpox and polio under control. People with diabetes can live long and healthy life, because of insulin injections. Antibiotics can overcome bacterial infections. Organ transplants can extend lives. Sophisticated diagnostic tools—x-rays, CAT scans, MRIs—can accurately detect disease.

But the focus of Western medicine is on the *treatment* of disease. We believe it is time to also focus on the *prevention* of disease. And there are some systems of healing that have done just that—for thousands of years.

One of them is traditional Chinese medicine (TCM). It looks primarily at the *person*, considering disease the result of an imbalance of physical, emotional, mental, and spiritual energies collectively called *chi*, or life-force.

The modalities of TCM include sophisticated diagnostic techniques based on the senses (such as pulse and tongue diagnosis), dietary therapy, herbal medicine, acupuncture, and massage. And in the best of circumstances, these modalities are used to detect imbalances early and correct them, preventing disease.

Recent research conducted by Dr. Bryan shows that some of the herbs used in TCM to both prevent and treat heart disease are uniquely rich in nitrate and nitrite—and uniquely powerful in generating NO in the body.

For the study, Dr. Bryan and his colleagues first went to a local oriental herb and acupuncture shop in Texas and bought herbs commonly used in TCM to treat heart disease: *DanShen*, *GauLou*, *XieBai*, and six others.

Next, they tested each herb three ways: (1) the herb's quantity of nitrate and nitrite, chemical precursors of NO production; (2) the herb's ability to generate nitric oxide from nitrate and nitrite; and (3) the herb's ability to

Listen to Joyful Music, Watch Funny Movies

In a study by researchers in the Division of Cardiology at the University of Maryland Medical Center, 10 people were asked to listen to either joy- or anxiety-provoking music, and then researchers measured the flow-mediated dilation—the amount their arteries widened, a sign of increased NO.

Joyful music increased flow-mediated dilation by 2.7 percent (the same amount as seen in exercise or after taking a cholesterol-lowering statin drug), whereas anxiety-producing music decreased it by 0.6 percent.

"Listening to joyful music may be an adjunctive life-style intervention for the promotion of vascular health," concluded the researchers in the journal *Psychosomatic Medicine*.

You might want to watch joyful movies, too.

In a similar study, 19 out of 20 people who watched a movie that made them laugh (such as the comedy *There's Something About Mary*) had an increase in flow-mediated dilation, whereas 14 of 20 people who watched stress-inducing movie clips (such as a realistic battle scene in the movie *Saving Private Ryan*) had a reduction in flow-mediated dilation. "Positive emotions such as mirthful laughter" have a positive effect on the endothelium, concluded the researchers in the medical journal *Heart*.

relax the blood vessels of laboratory animals by stimulating the production of NO in the endothelium.

The herbs were outstanding in all three areas.

They contained lots of nitrate and nitrite. They were able to turn those compounds into nitric oxide—in fact, one herb did it at a level a thousand times greater than the body does it. And they were very effective at relaxing and widening blood vessels through NO production. The findings were in the journal *Free Radical Biology and Medicine*.

Bottom line: traditional Chinese medicines that have been used for thousands of years have profound NO bioactivity. The herbs supply the NO precursors nitrate and nitrite. They generate NO from those precursors.

They restore the ability of the endothelium to produce NO. And they help preserve NO in the body, so its effects are long-lasting.

Scientific evidence linking TCM and NO

Many other recent studies make the connection between TCM and NO:

More proof of the NO-boosting power of Chinese herbs. Noting that "the purported effects of 'circulation-improving' herbs in TCM show striking similarities with the vascular action of nitric oxide produced by the endothelial NO synthase (eNOS)," German researchers tested the eNOS-boosting power of 15 herbs used in TCM to protect and heal the heart. They found that one of them—*Prunella vulgaris*, or Heal-All—was particularly powerful in producing eNOS and triggering its activity. In previous research, the scientists had found NO-increasing activity from *Dan Shen* (an herb also tested by Dr. Bryan in his study).

The NO-boosting power of Tongxinluo. Cardiologists at the Peking Union Medical College and the China Academy of Chinese Medical Sciences found that *Tongxinluo*—a traditional Chinese herb used for heart disease—works in part by generating eNOS, the enzyme in the endothelium that triggers the production of NO. The results were in the *American Journal of Physiology: Heart and Circulatory Physiology*.

TCM helps lowers high blood pressure—and increases NO. Researchers at the China Academy of Chinese Medical Sciences in Beijing treated 241 people with high blood pressure with either (1) *Jiangya*, a TCM herb traditionally used to improve circulation and lower blood pressure; (2) the herb *and* conventional pressure-lowering medication, or (3) the medication only. The herb/drug combination was the most effective—and while it was lowering blood pressure, it was boosting blood levels of NO.

Acupuncture raises NO. In an animal study, Chinese researchers found that electro-acupuncture (a form of the therapy that delivers a mild electrical current to acupuncture points) increased eNOS in rats with experimentally induced high blood pressure. The results were in the journal *Experimental Biology and Medicine*.

In another experiment, researchers at the China Academy of Chinese Medical Sciences studied 40 people, giving half acupuncture. After the treatment, they measured the level of NO at acupuncture points—and NO was "strikingly higher" at the acupuncture points compared to other spots on the skin. "Acupuncture stimulation can upregulate dermal [skin] NO content," concluded the researchers.

In fact, acupuncture may work *because* of NO on the skin, theorize researchers in the David Geffen School of Medicine at UCLA. They noted their animal and human research has shown:

- NO is increased in skin acupoints.
- Stimulating acupoints increases NO in brain cells.
- When NO is boosted with L-arginine, there is more electrical conductivity over acupoints.
- Giving animals a compound that boosts NO on the skin also boosts nerve activity at acupoints.
- In people, NO levels are much higher at acupoints than at other places on the skin.
- Using antibacterial products decreases NO on the skin.

Their conclusion: bacteria reduce nitrate on the skin, which generates NO on acupoints (and additional NO in the brain). Both sources of NO boost nerve activity at acupoints—which may be one major reason why acupuncture works! Another team of experts has a different perspective.

"Several studies have shown that acupuncture enhances the generation of NO and increases local circulation," commented Taiwanese researchers at the National Research Institute of Chinese Medicine, in a paper in the *Journal of Acupuncture and Meridian Studies*. But *how* does acupuncture do it? Their theory: the stimulus of acupuncture creates a "mechanical force transfer" from connective tissue to the "extracellular matrix" . . . which affects cells in the area . . . inducing the production of NO . . . which in turn "increases blood flow and local circulation."

Well, *however* acupuncture works to boost NO—we're glad it does. And if you're depressed, you might be glad, too.

Acupuncture can relieve depression—by lifting NO levels. That was the conclusion of another group of scientists at the China Academy of Chinese Medical Sciences. They used three weeks of stress and isolation to create a depression-like state in rats, while giving half the rats daily electro-acupuncture (EA). The rats receiving EA had much higher levels of nitric oxide synthase in their brain cells (nNOS) than the non-EA rats, as well as higher levels of another compound that sparks the production of NO (cGMP). "Electroacupuncture can upregulate the expression of nNOS and the content of cGMP" in the brains of depressed rats, "which may contribute to its effect in relieving depression," concluded the researchers.

Ear acupressure relieves menstrual symptoms—and increases NO. You can also stimulate acupuncture points with *finger pressure*—a technique called acupressure. Researchers from Taiwan studied 71 college students with menstrual cramps, teaching half of them acupressure, which they used for 20 days before their period. The technique decreased the pain during the next period by 86 percent compared to previous periods—and increased NO levels. The findings were in the *Journal of Alternative and Complementary Medicine*.

Moxibustion raises NO. In this technique from TCM, an herb (usually *moxa*, or mugwort) is safely burned over an acupuncture point. (The herb is removed before the flame ever touches the skin.) Doctors at the College of Chinese Medicine studied 209 women with menstrual cramps, giving half of them moxibustion treatments, and measuring blood levels of NO in both groups. The treatment was very effective in relieving cramps—and "considerably" increased NO. "Moxibustion is effective in relieving" menstrual cramps, wrote the researchers, concluding that this effect "may be closely associated" with its ability to raise blood NO.

· PART THREE ·

The New Science of NO

SIX

Is NO a No-No?

The Scientific Truth about the
Supposed Dangers of NO, Nitrate, and Nitrite

If you started reading this book at the beginning and read straight through to this chapter, you know that we've spent a lot of time making much of the health-preserving and health-restoring power of NO, urging you to boost your body's levels of the molecule in many different ways, including a diet rich in nitrate and nitrite.

But maybe you're saying to yourself, "Wait a second . . ."

Haven't I heard just the *opposite* about nitric oxide, nitrate, and nitrite—that they're *bad* for me?

Isn't nitric oxide a pollutant—one of the acids in acid rain, and one of the molecules that gave the Marlboro Man lung cancer?

And aren't nitrate and nitrite harmful food additives that play a role in the formation of N-nitrosamines, chemicals that cause cancer?

Well, those are good questions. And in this chapter we've tried to provide good answers.

Let's start with this observation: we're in the middle of a scientific revolution regarding nitric oxide (NO), nitrate, and nitrite.

The first stage in that revolution was the surprising (and even shocking) discovery (leading to a Nobel Prize) that NO—rather than being just a poisonous gas—was a crucial signaling molecule in the body, involved in the health of every tissue, organ, and system.

The second stage was the equally surprising discovery that NO was not only created by a pathway involving the amino acid L-arginine, but that NO levels in the body also depend on the presence of dietary nitrate and nitrite. (Both compounds are found in the diet, but nitrate is far more common. Nitrate then turns into nitrite in the body, which turns into NO. This process is discussed at length in Chapter 3.)

Like all revolutions in scientific understanding, it's taking time for these new findings to penetrate the entrenched perspectives about NO, nitrate, and nitrite.

But for the sake of our health, NO must claim its rightful place as a miracle molecule—a compound that can literally save your life.

For the same reason, nitrate and nitrite must be understood for what they truly are: essential nutrients that are keys to good health, and *not* cancer-causing threats.

This chapter is all about clearing up the misconceptions surrounding NO, nitrate, and nitrite. We'll discuss NO first, followed by nitrate and nitrite.

NO: Too Much of a Good Thing?

As you've read throughout this book, too *little* NO can cause all kinds of health problems, including high blood pressure, heart disease, and stroke.

But as Paracelsus, the famous physician of the Renaissance, wrote, "Poison is in everything, and no thing is without poison. The dosage makes it a poison or a remedy."

For example, too much *water* can kill you—and water has killed marathoners who drank too much during a race.

A healthy level of the trace mineral selenium has been shown to dramatically lower the risk of cancer. But that healthy level is measured in *micrograms*. Ingesting even five milligrams a day—much less than the RDA for many other nutrients—can poison you, creating a condition called *selenosis*, with symptoms including fatigue, hair loss, brain damage, and (if you ingest enough) death.

The mineral iron also illustrates the Paracelsus "poison-in-everything" principle. If you're a young woman with iron deficiency, you can suffer all kinds of problems, including fatigue, headaches, cold hands and feet, and poor memory. But too much iron stored in the body of an older man can cause heart disease and cancer!

NO is not an exception to this natural phenomena. Too little can hurt you—a lot. Too much can hurt you—a lot. But if levels are just right, you're just fine.

But *how* can too much NO hurt you? Surprise—it's a free radical.

The helpful free radical

No doubt you've read about the molecular bad guys called *free radicals*. Here's how they do their dirty work.

As you probably remember from Chemistry 101, chemicals are composed of molecules, which are made of atoms. An atom has a couple of moving (and unmoving) parts. In the center is the nucleus. Around the nucleus are orderly rings consisting of positively charged particles called *protons* and negatively charged particles called *electrons*.

Electrons are atomic glue—they "bond" with other electrons, allowing atoms to form molecules. In your average atom, the ring closest to the nucleus is filled with two electrons, and the ring beyond that is filled with eight. When that outer ring is packed with all the electrons it can hold, the atom is satisfied, or what scientists call *inert*: it doesn't try to do anything.

However, when that outer ring is *missing* an electron—when there's a so-called *unpaired* electron—the atom is dissatisfied: it tries to find another electron, perhaps by bonding with another atom. In chemistry, this is called a *reaction*, and the atoms or molecules that participate in the reaction are called *reactive*.

A free radical is a molecule with an unpaired electron. Think of it as a "criminal" molecule that "attacks" a nearby atom and "steals" an electron. Well, the attacked atom that had its electron ripped off joins the gang, and becomes a free radical itself. It attacks another molecule—and so on.

This free radical crime spree is responsible for a process called *oxidation* (free radicals are also called *reactive oxygen species*, or ROS). Like sunlight (which sustains life on Earth *and* damages cells), oxidation is both crucial *and* harmful to cellular life. In fact, some scientists and medical experts think free radicals and unchecked oxidation is *the* key process underlying chronic disease and aging.

NO is a free radical—an unusual free radical. Because NO is both bad and good, depending on the circumstances.

In normal quantities, NO is good: a crucial signaling molecule, controlling the tightening and widening of every organ and tissue, from your arteries to your eyes. Throughout the body, it is the master of *homeostasis*—of balance and good health.

But when NO is overproduced (because of an infection, chronic inflammation, or other possible causes), it can wreak bodily havoc. The scientific literature includes thousands of studies measuring the toxic effects of excessive NO on various organ systems, and suggesting ways to control it.

Bottom line: in normal amounts, NO provides all the cellular *protection* that has been described throughout this book. But when there is too much NO, cellular *destruction* is the result.

When NO is "just right"

How do you maintain a "just right" level of NO? Refer to Chapters 3, 4, and 5! But, in brief, it's a *balanced* lifestyle. That includes:

- Eat a diet rich in nitrate-packed green leafy vegetables.
- Emphasize foods and beverages rich in polyphenols (such as dark chocolate, green tea, and red wine), which boost the body's production of NO.
- Drink plenty of water—hydration helps cells manufacture NO.
- Consider taking an NO-increasing supplement, particularly if you're over 40—because aging cuts down on the body's production of NO.
- Get regular, NO-producing exercise.
- Create a schedule and an environment that ensures you'll get enough NO-restoring sleep.
- Control NO-depleting stress, through deep breathing and other stress-reduction techniques.

And don't believe everything you hear about nitrate and nitrite!

Nitrate and Nitrite: Two Good Guys with (Undeserved) Bad Reputations

Once upon a scientific time, the "inorganic" (a chemical term) compounds nitrate and nitrite were thought to be inert: useless byproducts in the generation of the very useful NO.

They were also thought to be dangerous: possible cancer-causers that you should avoid if you could help it.

But time changes, including scientific times. Nitrate and nitrite are now understood to play a very active and key role in causing *health*, by helping to form NO in the body, and also by directly contributing to a strong, clean circulatory system.

Let's look at the developing understanding about these two compounds—and the persistent misunderstandings that need to be debunked.

The history of nitrate and nitrite

Nitrate and nitrite have been used for thousands of years as food preservatives, a process known as "curing"—*the* way to preserve meat before the advent of refrigeration. In the 19th century, it was discovered that nitrate works as a preservative by turning into nitrite, and food scientists starting using sodium nitrite as the primary preservative in meat. Nitrite works as a preservative in several ways. It:

- delays rancidity (the oxidation of fat) during storage.
- controls the growth of *Listeria monocytogenes*, a bacteria that can cause food poisoning, particularly in pregnant women.
- delays the development of the toxin *Clostridium botulinum* (botulism) in unrefrigerated meat.
- develops the color and flavor of cured meat (for you chemistry buffs out there: nitrite works to provide a red color to meat by reacting with oxymyoglobin to form S-nitrosomyoglobin).
- preserves the flavors of smoke and spice.
- inhibits the development of a "warmed-over" flavor in cured meat.

But the 1950s and 1960s saw the beginnings of concern about the use of nitrite in meat. It was discovered that nitrite (and nitrate) could cause *nitrosation* of *amines* (a molecule containing a nitrogen atom), creating N-nitrosamines, compounds that might be carcinogenic.

In 1964, it was discovered that such reactions could occur in food—specifically, in nitrite-preserved fish.

In 1969, scientists showed the same reaction could occur in the human stomach.

And so, by the 1970s, there was a major public health concern about nitrite in foods: were processed meats carcinogenic, because of their propensity to generate N-nitrosamines? We think the answer is no. But plenty of other scientists thought, and continue to think, that the answer is yes. Let's look at the science behind their opinion.

The epidemiological evidence

One way scientists investigate a link between a so-called *risk factor* in food and a specific disease is to conduct an *epidemiological study*. This research typically focuses on a specific health habit (such as the consumption of meat processed with nitrite) and correlates it with a specific disease (such as cancer). If a link is found between the habit and the disease, epidemiologists don't claim the habit *caused* the disease. Rather, they say they have discovered an *association*—a possible link—between the two.

(It takes many additional types of studies to prove that an epidemiological association is an actual cause of disease: animal studies to see if the risk factor actually causes harm in a living being; if it does cause harm, mechanistic and metabolic studies to figure out *why* it causes harm; and clinical studies to find out if what is true in animals is also true in people.)

If epidemiologists find an increased risk, they call it by various names, such as "relative risk" and "hazard ratio." And they calculate it in various ways. For example, they might say the "relative risk" was increased by 40 percent. Or they might express no risk as the number 1.0, and express the 40 percent increase as the number 1.4.

Well, if you enter the words "nitrate," "nitrite," and "cancer" into the database of the National Institutes of Health, you'll discover dozens of epidemiological studies exploring the link between those two compounds and cancer. We're going to report on a couple of the most recent studies—and then show you why they're so wrong-minded in their conclusion that nitrate and nitrite are threats to your health.

Thyroid cancer. Researchers from the National Cancer Institute (NCI) at the National Institutes of Health (NIH) analyzed diet and health data from nearly 500 thousand people, and found no link between nitrite intake and thyroid cancer. But they found a 2.28 (228 percent) greater risk in those who consumed the most dietary nitrate compared to those who consumed the least. The findings were in the *International Journal of Cancer.*

Non-Hodgkin lymphoma (NHL). The same team of NCI researchers looked at a group of 1,304 women, and didn't find an increased risk for this blood cancer among women with the highest level of dietary nitrite intake. But they did find a so-called "significant" link between high nitrite intake and some subtypes of lymphoma, such as follicular lymphoma and T-cell lymphoma. The findings were in the medical journal *Cancer Causes and Control.*

Prostate cancer. In a nine-year study of nearly 200 thousand men, the NCI researchers found a 1.07 (7 percent) greater risk for prostate cancer among men who ate the most processed meat. And they found an increased risk for advanced prostate cancer among men with the highest intake of nitrate (1.31, or 31 percent) and nitrite (1.24, or 24 percent). The findings were in the *American Journal of Epidemiology.*

Colorectal cancer. More research from the NCI: in a study of more than 300 thousand people, the researchers found those with the highest intake of nitrate from processed meats had a 1.16 (16 percent) increased risk of colorectal cancer. The findings were in the journal *Cancer Research.*

Brain cancer. A team of UK researchers found no increased risk for glioma (a type of brain tumor) among those with the highest intake of processed meats compared to those with the lowest intake. (In fact, they find a slightly decreased risk.) They found a 1.02 (2 percent) greater risk for glioma among those with the highest consumption of nitrate; and a 1.26 greater risk (26 percent) among those with the highest consumption of nitrite. The findings were in the *American Journal of Clinical Nutrition.*

Bladder cancer. In a study of more than 300 thousand people, the NCI researchers found that those with the highest intake of nitrite had a 1.28

(28 percent) increased risk for bladder cancer, and those with the highest intake of nitrate and nitrite from processed meats had a 1.29 (29 percent) increased risk. The findings were in the journal *Cancer*.

What do all those results *mean*, in terms of what you should and shouldn't eat?

Well, in a summary report, the World Cancer Research Fund and the American Institute for Cancer Research presented a recommendation to "avoid processed meats," based on a meta-analysis of studies that showed a link between processed meats and colorectal cancer—with an increased risk of 1.21 (21 percent) for every 50 grams (1.8 ounces) per day of consumption.

(A lengthy aside before continuing the discussion of nitrate and nitrite: we think that's an extreme recommendation. When you try to "avoid" any food—when you forbid yourself a food, whether it's a slice of bacon or a banana split—you usually end up bingeing on it. Not only that, red meat—including processed meat—can supply an important share of vital nutrients in a normal diet. A better recommendation: you should *maximize* your intake of whole foods such as vegetables, fruits, fish, beans, whole grains, and nuts and seeds, and *minimize* your intake of cured and processed meats such as ham, bacon, hot dogs, corned beef, lunch meats, and sausages, enjoying them every now and then, if you want to. You should also minimize your intake of saturated fat from red meat and full-fat dairy products, and minimize your intake of refined carbohydrates such as sugar and white flour. That's a sensible recommendation that's workable in the real world. Now, back to nitrate and nitrite . . .)

Does the fact that processed meats might (and that's a really big *might*) increase your risk for cancer mean you should avoid nitrate and nitrite in food, because they're supposedly cancer-causers?

That's exactly the conclusion reached by many nutritionists.

We think that idea is dead wrong. In fact, we think it's so wrong you could end up dead!

Dr. Bryan was (and is) so concerned about this mistaken point of view that he was moved to counter it by cowriting a scientific paper on the topic, publishing it in the journal *Nitric Oxide*. It's titled (in the precise phrasing favored by scientists): "Nutritional epidemiology in the context of nitric oxide biology: A risk-benefit evaluation for dietary nitrite and nitrate." Here are Dr. Bryan's counter-arguments for those who say nitrate and nitrite put your health at risk.

The association is weak

As you probably noticed, the "association" between a high intake of nitrate and nitrite—if it was found to exist at all—is typically not a strong one. Most of the increased risk was on the level of 1.2, 1.3, or 1.4. (By comparison, the relative risk of smokers developing lung cancer is 10 times higher—10.0—than nonsmokers.)

Epidemiologists call such an association *weak*. In 1994, the National Cancer Institute said that "relative risks" below 2.0 (200 percent) were not strong enough to make public policy pronouncements about risk factors.

Nitrate and nitrite are not the only "risky" compounds in processed meat

When looking at studies that find an association between the intake of cured meats and cancer, it's important to remember that nitrate and nitrite are only two among many bioactive compounds in those meats. Some of the studies we just reported looked at other meat-related compounds and even meat-related lifestyle factors, including: red meat itself, saturated fat, heme iron (the type of iron found in meat), benzopyrene (a compound formed when meat is cooked), heterocyclic amines (a compound formed when meat is deep fried or grilled), and grilling and barbecuing itself—and they *all* increased risk to one degree or another! So, is the risk from *one* of those factors? From a *few* of them? From *all* of them, and only when they're found together? No one really knows. And it's nearly impossible to know.

Are vegetables carcinogens?

Needless to say, dietary nitrate and nitrite isn't only found in cured meat. These compounds are also found in vegetables. Is broccoli a carcinogen? Is kale? Spinach? The epidemiological research that we discussed in Chapter 3 shows just the opposite: these foods are linked to the *prevention* of cancer.

A telling point: a person eating a vegetable-rich DASH diet to lower high blood pressure has an intake of nitrate *five times higher* than the "acceptable daily intake" proposed by the World Health Organization because of their concern nitrate is a carcinogen. This type of illogic is typical of the official thinking around nitrate and nitrite.

Is your saliva carcinogenic?

If nitrite is a carcinogen, we should all stop swallowing our own saliva—now! That's because saliva contains a goodly amount of nitrite, which increases after a nitrate-rich meal, such as a spinach salad. Yet studies involving thousands of people have failed to find any evidence for a link between nitrate intake and stomach cancer—a link that should be obvious if the dietary nitrate and nitrite in saliva were carcinogens.

Another telling point: normal levels of nitrate and nitrite in saliva and the rest of your body are much higher than amounts considered by health authorities to put your health at risk!

Why aren't more Tibetans dying of cancer?

Studies on people in Tibet who live at high altitudes showed that increased levels of nitrate and nitrite in their bodies (100 times higher than people living at sea level in America!) are *natural physiological oxygen-boosting responses* to the low levels of oxygen in the atmosphere—and completely free of any harmful effects. Tibetans don't have any nitrate- or nitrite-caused illnesses. And they don't have a higher rate of cancer. If nitrate and nitrite were carcinogens, they'd be dying of cancer in droves.

Five thousand years of Phase 1 safety trials

As we described in Chapter 5, many of the herbs used to treat heart disease in traditional Chinese medicine (TCM) are very high in nitrate and also contain nitrite. And in animal studies these herbs generate high levels of nitric oxide. TCM has been used to protect and improve health for five thousand years, with no record of its herbal treatments causing cancer. In fact, we're confident that if these nitrate-rich herbs had any harmful effects, they would have been recognized long ago.

In essence, Phase 1 safety trials of nitrate and nitrite—the type of study conducted by a drug company to ensure that the medication it is bringing to market is safe—have been conducted for the past five thousand years.

Who put the nitrate and nitrite in breast milk!?!

One of the most compelling arguments for the *requirement* for nitrate and nitrite in the diet is the fact that these two compounds appear in high levels in the breast milk of newly nursing mothers, imparting both nutritional and immunological benefits to the baby. In fact, tests show that the breast milk of newly nursing mothers contains *more* nitrite than any other food or beverage!

If nitrate and nitrite are carcinogens, what are they doing in breast milk? They're *not* carcinogens. They're there to keep the baby healthy. Here's what's happening:

The production of health-giving NO in the body requires the presence of NO-producing bacteria in the saliva and the digestive tract that turn nitrite into NO. In newborns, those bacteria haven't fully colonized the body. To make up for the difference—to make sure NO is produced—Mother Nature provides nitrate and nitrite in breast milk. As the baby grows, and its body is colonized with NO-producing bacteria, levels of nitrate and nitrite in breast milk decrease.

Bizarrely enough, the World Health Organization has set the acceptable daily intake of nitrate and nitrite per kilogram of body weight *lower* than what is required by an infant from breast milk!

(This discrepancy is a glaring example of the wrong understanding about these two compounds that is still prevalent within the nutritional and scientific communities.)

If there were *any* merit to the contention that nitrate and nitrite promote cancer, we would see a higher incidence of cancer in breast-fed babies compared to formula-fed babies (formula has lower levels of nitrate and nitrite than mother's milk). But there's no such difference.

Mother Nature has devised a perfect system to nourish and foster the growth and development of nursing babies—and it looks like nitrite is an indispensable nutrient in that system.

A few words about N-nitrosamines

One of the biggest concerns about nitrate and nitrite is their ability to form the carcinogens called N-nitrosamines and cause stomach cancer.

There are many ways to be exposed to the more than 300 N-nitrosamine

The Blue Baby Syndrome: Is Nitrite to Blame?

The level of nitrate in drinking water is regulated by the government, but not because of a concern for cancer.

The reason: in infants under six months of age, exposure to excess nitrate in well water contaminated with bacteria (which turns nitrate into nitrite) is thought to cause *methemoglobinemia*, or "blue baby syndrome"—nitrite oxidizes the iron in oxygen-carrying hemoglobin, and adequate oxygen can't get to tissues, causing the baby's skin to turn blue (and causing other health problems as well).

Because nitrite is seen as the guilty party in methemoglobinemia, an American Academy of Pediatrics consensus panel declared that home-prepared (not commercial) baby food from nitrite-containing vegetables such as spinach, beets, green beans, squash, and carrots shouldn't be fed to an infant until the child is at least 3-months old.

But are nitrate and nitrite *really* the cause of blue baby syndrome?

A wide range of studies in which children and adults have been given big doses of nitrate and nitrite didn't produce methemoglobinemia. In the latest development, scientists are proposing other reasons for the problem, such as a bacterial infection of the stomach (gastroenteritis), or the overproduction of NO because of bacterial invasion. But not because of the nitrate and nitrite.

Yes, the *theory* that nitrite toxicity causes methemoglobinemia is plausible. But this plausible hypothesis has become a dogma—in spite of the lack of proof that it is correct.

carcinogens—through diet, tobacco products, cosmetics, medications, agricultural chemicals, and occupational exposure (such as the manufacturing of tires and other rubber products).

The main dietary source: fried bacon, because at the high temperatures of frying the amines in meat form N-nitrosamines. They're also formed in an acid environment, such as the stomach.

But the formation of N-nitrosamines from dietary nitrate and nitrite is far from automatic. You have to have amines—and there are very small amounts of amines in meat, most of which are *primary amines* that don't form N-nitrosamine. You have to heat the meat above 266°F (frying or grilling will do it). And you have to have a low pH (high acid) environment.

Two more important points.

Vitamin C and other antioxidants are routinely added to bacon, and they dramatically reduce the formation of N-nitrosamines.

And there is very little evidence showing that N-nitrosamines actually cause cancer in humans.

It's not that N-nitrosamines aren't a concern; they are. Eat bacon as an occasional treat rather than daily.

It's that the dietary nitrate and nitrite that play a role in the formation of N-nitrosamines are *not* a health concern, for all the reasons we've discussed.

Where's the beef?

That catch phrase became wildly popular after a Wendy's commercial in which an elderly woman looked inside the hamburger bun of a competing fast food chain and complained about the lack of meat. Well, there's very little "beef" to the link between nitrate, nitrite, and cancer—that is, very little direct evidence of the carcinogenicity of nitrate and nitrite, in spite of 40 years of intense investigation.

As Dr. Bryan wrote, citing a paper from a researcher from the National Cancer Institute: "A causative and specific link between nitrate or nitrite exposure and cancer is still missing."

In fact, a two-year state-of-the-art animal study on the carcinogenicity of sodium nitrite by the NIH found no conclusive evidence of carcinogenic activity.

In California, a review of 99 studies on sodium nitrite led the state's Developmental and Reproductive Toxicant Identification Committee of eight independent scientists to conclude that sodium nitrite should *not* be listed under California's Proposition 65 law, which requires the state to identify chemicals that can cause cancer and birth defects.

And a study from Swiss researchers, in the journal *Nutrition Reviews*, declared: "Epidemiologic evidence of the carcinogenic potential of dietary [N-nitrosamines] and precursor nitrates and nitrites in humans remains inconclusive with regard to the risk of stomach, brain, esophageal, and nasopharyngeal cancers."

The New Understanding of Nitrate and Nitrite

In the late 1970s—in spite of all the fear and paranoia surrounding nitrite exposure—the scientific understanding of and appreciation for nitrate and nitrite took a dramatic turn.

First, studies found that nitrate and nitrite—supposed carcinogens—are actually *formed* in the intestinal tract. (This discovery eventually lead to the discovery of the L-arginine-NO pathway, discussed earlier in the book.) Before this, it was thought that levels of nitrate and nitrite in the body were *only* from dietary sources, and from bacteria. Since this discovery, it's understood that nitrate and nitrite are *natural* molecules, produced by *normal* metabolism.

As research progressed, many more findings were made about the role of nitrate and nitrite in health, mostly from animal studies.

Helping out in heart failure. Nitrite can form NO during heart failure, protecting the heart from injury.

Limiting tissue damage in disease. Supplying nitrite to an oxygen-deprived tissue or organ can limit the amount of damage to the area (such as after transplantation surgery, heart attack, or stroke).

Storing NO. Nitrite is a major storage form of NO in tissues—in fact, nitrite is an excellent biomarker of NO levels. Increase NO in the body, and you increase nitrite. Increase nitrite in the body, and you increase NO.

Improving blood flow. Nitrite increases blood flow and oxygen delivery to tissues, just like NO.

Reducing injury. Nitrite has shown a remarkable ability to reduce injury from heart attack, liver damage, kidney damage, stroke, and spasms of the blood vessels in the brain.

Lowering blood pressure. If nitrite is given orally, it can effectively restore NO levels and lower high blood pressure.

Cooling inflammation. Nitrite also decreases inflammation and reduces levels of C-reactive protein (a biomarker for artery-damaging inflammation).

Helping in sickle cell anemia. Nitrite can increase blood flow in people with sickle cell anemia.

The Nitrogen Cycle: Nature Likes Nitrate and Nitrite

Earth's atmosphere is 78 percent nitrogen. But that nitrogen is chemically inert—animals and plants can't use it—and it's converted into other compounds, such as nitrate and nitrite. That conversion is done mainly by bacteria, which take nitrogen from the air and perform the chemical magic known as "nitrogen fixation"—nitrogen becomes ammonium, and ammonium becomes nitrate and nitrite. The plants use the nitrate for food and fertilizer. In generating those compounds, the bacteria get the nutrients they need (and a nice place to live). When you eat the nitrate in a plant, the friendly bacteria in your body go to work, transforming it into nitrite, which is then transformed into heart-saving NO.

Nature doesn't have any mistaken ideas about the importance of nitrogen—and nitrate and nitrite—to life (and health) on Earth.

Boosted by exercise. Like NO, blood levels of nitrite increase after exercise in healthy people (whereas in older people with endothelial dysfunction, there's no increase in nitrite).

Nitrite and fitness. Nitrite levels in the blood are also predictive of a person's exercise capacity.

Because of these studies, there are now many more studies testing nitrate and nitrite in people—healthy people, and people with heart disease.

Bottom line: nitrate and nitrite have very important and crucial functions in the body—including providing a backup system for the production of NO, as we discussed at length in Chapter 3.

It's time for a reevaluation of the nitrate and nitrite in our diets. The strategy from the 1970s of *limiting* nitrate- and nitrite-rich foods because they might form N-nitrosamines is not justified—and may be dangerous to your heart's health!

A new understanding of the *health-creating* (and NO-creating) power of nitrate and nitrite must be established and communicated to experts and to the public.

As Dr. Bryan wrote in his paper on nitrate and nitrite: "It is time for health care professionals, clinical nutritionists, dieticians, food scientists and epidemiologists to begin discussion and appreciate contemporary views of nitrite and nitrate as *indispensable nutrients.*"

Is nitrite a new vitamin?

In a report from the National Research Council, it was estimated that the average daily intake of nitrate and nitrite in the US is 76 mg and 0.77 mg, respectively. If we assume the average person produces about 76 mg of nitrite internally (a reasonable estimate from what we now know about the physiology of this compound), we can see that about *half* of the nitrite in our daily lives is from the diet. (That's just another hole in the logic of identifying nitrite as a carcinogen.)

In fact, the emerging data on dietary nitrite makes it look like it's very similar to a vitamin.

By definition, a vitamin is: any one of a group of organic substances essential in small quantities for health, found in small quantities in natural foods, or sometimes produced within the body (such as vitamin K, produced by intestinal bacteria). Deficiencies of vitamins produce specific illnesses.

Nitrite meets those criteria.

It's found in minute quantities in natural foods and also produced in the body during normal metabolism.

And could it be that if you don't eat enough nitrite-forming nitrate, specific disorders occur?

We would say yes—specifically, cardiovascular disease! And perhaps many other diseases as well.

In fact, this entire book is purposed to let you know about the importance of NO, and its precursors nitrate and nitrite, and how to increase your intake and production of these life-saving factors.

We hope this chapter has allayed any fears you might have had about doing just that!

About the Authors

Nathan S. Bryan, PhD

Dr. Nathan S. Bryan is an assistant professor of molecular medicine within the Brown Foundation Institute of Molecular Medicine, part of the School of Medicine at the University of Texas Health Science Center at Houston. He is also on faculty within the Department of Integrative Biology and Pharmacology and Graduate School of Biomedical Sciences at the UT Houston Medical School. Dr. Bryan earned his undergraduate Bachelor of Science degree in Biochemistry from the University of Texas at Austin and his doctoral degree from Louisiana State University School of Medicine in Shreveport, where he was the recipient of the Dean's Award for Excellence in Research. He pursued his postdoctoral training as a Kirschstein Fellow at Boston University School of Medicine in the Whitaker Cardiovascular Institute. Dr. Bryan joined the Institute of Molecular Medicine, University of Texas Health Science Center at Houston, in June 2006 in the Center for Cell Signaling. He is an active member of the Nitric Oxide Society, Society for Free Radical Biology and Medicine, and the American Heart Association.

Dr. Bryan's research is dedicated to providing a better understanding of the interactions of nitric oxide and related metabolites with their different biological targets at the molecular and cellular levels, and the significance of these reactions for physiology and pathophysiology. Attempts are made to identify what particular changes in NO-related signaling pathways and reaction products occur in disease states such as endothelial dysfunction, ischemia/reperfusion, tissue/cardiac protection, diabetes, atherosclerosis, and inflammation, with the aim of testing their amenability as biomarkers for diagnosis and/or treatment of specific disease. Current research is directed to understanding the interactions of exogenous dietary nitrate/nitrite (NOx) on the endogenous NO/cGMP pathway, and how perturbations in each system affect cardiovascular health.

Dr. Bryan and colleagues recently discovered that nitrite is a biologically active molecule that was previously thought to be an inert breakdown product of NO production. These findings have unveiled many beneficial effects of nitrite in the treatment and prevention of human disease. These discoveries may provide the basis for new preventive or therapeutic strategies in diseases associated with NO insufficiency, and new guidelines for optimal health. Dr. Bryan has published a number of highly cited papers and authored or edited four books.

Dr. Bryan currently resides in Houston with his wife Kristen and their three sons, Grant, Lincoln, and Conley. The Bryans spend their weekends at their ranch near Caldwell, where they raise cattle and horses and enjoy the great outdoors. Nathan enjoys playing golf, as well as calf roping and team roping on his ranch and in competition.

Janet Zand, OMD

Dr. Janet Zand, L.Ac., OMD, Dipl. Ac., Dipl. CH., was the cofounder and Chairman of the Board of ZAND Herbal Formulas, Inc., from 1978 to 2002. ZAND Herbal Formulas was an industry pioneer. The company spent over 20 years as a market leader in the herbal industry. Dr. Zand's original, clinically based formula, Insure Herbal, was the first popular Echinacea/Goldenseal formula in the United States. Shortly thereafter, ZAND introduced Female and Male Formulas, becoming the first American company to combine Western and traditional Chinese herbs for the consumer. ZAND continued for more than 20 years to satisfy the growing consumer interest in natural alternatives to pharmaceutical medicines. ZAND produced over 100 formulas, which combined potent key ingredients with a blend of supportive herbs to restore and maintain the body's natural state of balance.

Dr. Zand has over 25 years of private practice experience in acupuncture, herbal medicine, homeopathy, and nutrition. She received a Bachelor of Arts degree from Sarah Lawrence College, and a Doctor of Oriental Medicine degree from California Acupuncture College. She is a Diplomate of Acupuncture and Chinese Herbs.

Dr. Zand is the author of several books, including *Smart Medicine for a Healthier Child* (Avery, 1994), *A Parent's Guide to Medical Emergencies* (Avery, 1997), and *Smart Medicine for a Healthier Living* (Avery, 1998). She has authored and been interviewed for multiple articles for more than two dozen publications including *Journal of Alternative Medicine*, *Cosmopolitan*, the *Wall Street Journal*, the *New York Times*, the *Los Angeles Times*, *Men's Fitness Magazine*, and *Allure*.

Dr. Zand currently serves on the Biomedicine Board for the National Certification Commission for Acupuncture and Oriental Medicine.

Bill Gottlieb

Bill Gottlieb is a book author and journalist, specializing in health, and the editorial director of the book packaging company Good For You Books.

Gottlieb worked for 20 years at Rodale, Inc., as associate editor, senior editor, and assistant managing editor of *Prevention Magazine*, as managing editor and executive editor of Prevention Magazine Health books, and as editor-in-chief and senior vice-president of Rodale Books.

Gottlieb became a freelance author and journalist in 1997. His articles have appeared in many past and present national periodicals, including Prevention, Reader's Digest, Bottom Line/Personal, Bottom Line/Health, Health, Cosmopolitan, Self, Men's Health, Runner's World, Natural Solutions, Organic Gardening, Best Life, Natural Health, and Bottom Line/ Women's Health.

As an author, his books have sold more than two million copies, and have been translated into Spanish, Chinese, and Arabic. They include: *Alternative Cures* (Rodale, 2000; Ballantine, 2008); *The Calcium Key*, with Michael Zemel, PhD (Wiley, 2004); *The DERMAdoctor Skinstruction Manual*, with Audrey Kunin, MD (Simon & Schuster, 2005); *The Natural Fat-Loss Pharmacy*, with Harry Preuss, MD (Broadway, 2007); *Breakthroughs in Drug-Free Healing* (Bottom Line Books, 2008); *Speed Healing* (Bottom Line Books, 2009); *Bottom Line's Breakthroughs in Natural Healing, 2011* (Bottom Line Books, 2010); and *The Real Cause, The Real Cure*, with Jacob Teitelbaum, MD (Rodale, 2011).

Index